W9-DFQ-209

e-Prescribing

e-Prescribing
The Electronic Transformation of Medicine

Jack E. Fincham, PhD, RPh
Professor
Department of Pharmacy Practice and Administration
University of Missouri–Kansas City

JONES AND BARTLETT PUBLISHERS
Sudbury, Massachusetts
BOSTON   TORONTO   LONDON   SINGAPORE

World Headquarters

Jones and Bartlett Publishers	Jones and Bartlett Publishers	Jones and Bartlett Publishers
40 Tall Pine Drive	Canada	International
Sudbury, MA 01776	6339 Ormindale Way	Barb House, Barb Mews
978-443-5000	Mississauga, Ontario L5V 1J2	London W6 7PA
info@jbpub.com	Canada	United Kingdom
www.jbpub.com		

Jones and Bartlett's books and products are available through most bookstores and online booksellers. To contact Jones and Bartlett Publishers directly, call 800-832-0034, fax 978-443-8000, or visit our website at www.jbpub.com.

Substantial discounts on bulk quantities of Jones and Bartlett's publications are available to corporations, professional associations, and other qualified organizations. For details and specific discount information, contact the special sales department at Jones and Bartlett via the above contact information or send an email to specialsales@jbpub.com.

Copyright © 2009 by Jones and Bartlett Publishers, LLC

All rights reserved. No part of the material protected by this copyright notice may be reproduced or utilized in any form, electronic or mechanical, including photocopying, recording, or any information storage or retrieval system, without written permission from the copyright owner.

Production Credits
Publisher: David Cella
Editorial Assistant: Maro Asadoorian
Production Manager: Julie Champagne Bolduc
Production Assistant: Jessica Steele Newfell
Associate Marketing Manager: Lisa Gordon
Manufacturing and Inventory Control Supervisor: Amy Bacus
Composition: Cape Cod Compositors, Inc.
Cover Design: Brian Moore
Cover Images: © Photos.com
Printing and Binding: Malloy, Inc.
Cover Printing: Malloy, Inc.

Library of Congress Cataloging-in-Publication Data
Fincham, Jack E.
E-prescribing : the electronic transformation of medicine / Jack E. Fincham.
p. ; cm.
Includes index.
ISBN 978-0-7637-5401-3 (pbk. : alk. paper)
1. Internet pharmacies. 2. Drugs—Prescribing—Data processing.
3. Pharmaceutical industry—Technological innovations. I. Title.
[DNLM: 1. Medical Order Entry Systems. 2. Prescriptions, Drug. QV 748 E48 2009]
RS122.2.F56 2009
381'.45615102854678—dc22   2008025966

6048

Printed in the United States of America
12 11 10 09 08   10 9 8 7 6 5 4 3 2 1

To Kelcie Jacqueline, the future Dr. Fincham.
Thank you for bringing so much joy and happiness so readily.

CONTENTS

PREFACE

Electronic prescribing (e-prescribing) holds the promise of revolutionizing how prescription medications are ordered, dispensed, and monitored. The confluence of many factors has highlighted with urgency the need to change how prescriptions are written, processed, dispensed, and monitored. As they unfold and mature, these factors will change the delivery of health care in the United States and beyond. Awareness of medical errors, federal and state governmental efforts to incorporate health information technology (IT), and changes in financing of health care and services have converged to focus private and public groups, associations, organizations, and consumer groups to change the drug prescribing process in the United States.

Medical Errors

Medical errors leading to harm due to drug name confusion, physician errors in transcribing brand names of drugs, and those mistakes resulting from physicians not recognizing the similarity of names of drugs can be effectively reduced by e-prescribing technology. Medical errors exact a tremendous toll on all associated with their occurrence. The National Coordinating Council for Medication Error Reporting and Prevention has defined a medical error as the following:[1]

> A medication error is any preventable event that may cause or lead to inappropriate medication use or patient harm while the medication is in the control of the healthcare professional, patient, or consumer. Such events may be related to professional practice, healthcare practice, healthcare products, procedures, and systems, including prescribing; order communication; product labeling, packaging, and nomenclature; compounding; dispensing; distribution; administration; education; monitoring and use.

Harm resulting from prescribing errors is a real concern for patients and all associated with their care. Harm has been defined by the United States Pharmacopeia (USP) as: "Impairment of the physical, emotional, or psychological function or structure of the body and/or pain resulting therefrom."[2]

Drug Name Similarity Confusion Leading to Errors and Harm

The USP analyzes various factors related to medication use in the United States. In the 2008 MEDMARX data report, USP chronicled a variety of medical errors due to using the wrong drug from drug name pairs with similar spelling and sounding trade names.[3] Using a nonproprietary name can reduce this cause of medical errors. Reinders notes in this report: "Reliance on the use of nonproprietary names is a starting point toward reducing medication errors that are associated with patient injury and death."[3(p.9)] One of the many alarming and interesting facets of the MEDMARX report is the analysis of sound-alike drug pairs and their occurrence over time. Cousins notes: "Together these sound-alike drug name pairs constituted more than 3,170 pairs—nearly double the 1,750 product pairs appearing on the 2004 list."[3(p.3)] This is not an innocuous concern; Cousins reports that 1.4% of errors associated with these sound-alike names led to the wrong drug being prescribed, resulting in patient harm.[3]

As detailed later in this book, e-prescribing will allow physicians and pharmacists to reduce medical errors due to drug name confusion by drug (both proprietary and nonproprietary drug) nomenclature software programs associated with e-prescribing software. Most importantly, patients will be the real beneficiary of medical error reductions attributable to e-prescribing.

Consumer-Driven Impact

There are more and more efforts in place allowing consumers to maintain their health records electronically. For example, WebMD[4] and iGuard[5] are but two of many companies or organizations that have enabled options for consumers to personally enter their drug therapy records online and have their medication taking monitored by others. Carrying this one step further, Google recently offered options for patients to load their medical records into cyberspace.[6] These consumer-driven efforts and options may provide an impetus for caregivers and providers to implement health IT and e-prescribing options sooner than expected.

Federal Government Efforts

As will be described in later chapters, the U.S. federal government has played a major role in fostering health IT implementation.[7]

Office of the National Coordinator for Health Information Technology

The Bush administration's institution of an Office of the National Coordinator for Health Information Technology (ONC) has prominently stimulated health IT awareness, including e-prescribing.

Private Consortia Efforts

The National Alliance for Health Information Technology (i.e., the Alliance) is an organization representing academic medical centers, hospitals, ambulatory care providers, integrated delivery networks, health systems, payors, purchasers, technology vendors, consultants, supply chain manufacturers and suppliers, associations, and other aligned stakeholders working to advance health care information technology.[8] The U.S. ONC has relied upon the Alliance to help standardize health IT terminology such as: electronic health record (EHR), electronic medical record (EMR), personal health record (PHR), health information exchange (HIE), and regional health information organization (RHIO).

Through comments submitted and consensus resulting from commentary periods, these terms will have a standard meaning as health IT adoption becomes ubiquitous. e-Prescribing terminology and architecture are imbedded in these efforts.

Centers for Medicare and Medicaid Services

Since November 2005, the Centers for Medicare and Medicaid Services (CMS) has published standards related to e-prescribing. The more efficient and speedy reimbursement opportunities offered by e-prescribing implementation will have an economic impact upon pharmacies. CMS encouragement and proposed mandates by 2009 requiring e-prescribing as a condition of participation has understandably boosted the importance of e-prescribing. Associated Medicare

Prescription Drug Plans (PDPs) and Medicare Advantage plans in the CMS Medicare Part D Drug Program that contract with pharmacy benefit management (PBM) companies have already benefited from e-prescribing implementation.

Physicians and physician office staff will reap time-saving and money-saving features of e-prescribing. Reducing the time-wasting callbacks to pharmacies to clarify prescription orders occurs readily after e-prescribing is adopted by medical offices.

As has been the case for decades, the U.S. private and public sectors institutionalize improvements of each entity's efforts regarding the medication use process.

Summary

I began this book with a desire to stay unbiased in my view of e-prescribing and the benefits, disadvantages, current state of uptake of the technology, and future opportunities. I hope you are able to learn from reading this book as much as I did in writing it.

References

1. National Coordinating Council for Medication Error Reporting and Prevention. *Homepage*. Available at: http://www.nccmerp.org. Accessed March 25, 2008.
2. United States Pharmacopeia. *Medication Errors Reporting Program*. Available at: http://www.usp.org/pdf/EN/patientSafety/medform.pdf. Accessed March 25, 2008.
3. Hicks RW, Becker SC, Cousins DD (eds). *MEDMARX Data Report: A Report on the Relationship of Drug Names and Medication Errors in Response to the Institute of Medicine's Call for Action*. Rockville, MD: Center for the Advancement of Patient Safety, U.S. Pharmacopeia; 2008.
4. WebMD. *Personal Health Record*. Available at: http://www.webmd.com/phr. Accessed March 25, 2008.
5. iGuard. *iGuard Homepage*. Available at: http://www.iguard.org. Accessed March 25, 2008.
6. Liston B. Google unveils personal medical record service. *Reuters*. February 28, 2008; Online. Available at: http://www.reuters.com/article/technologyNews/idUSN2854 822020080229. Accessed March 25, 2008.
7. National Alliance for Health Information Technology. *About NAHIT*. Available at: http://www.nahit.org/cms. Accessed March 25, 2008.
8. Centers for Medicare and Medicaid Studies. *e-Prescribing Overview*. Available at: http://www.cms.hhs.gov/EPrescribing. Accessed March 25, 2008.

NOTE TO READERS

As this book was going to press, two additional developments ensued that must be presented to the reader. One development is the merger of SureScripts and RxHub into SureScripts-RxHub. SureScripts forwards (routes) prescription information from prescribers to pharmacies while RxHub provides prescription eligibility, pharmacy benefit, drug formulary, and medication history information to physicians at the point of care. As noted on the SureScripts website, the July 1, 2008, merger details are as follows:[1]

> RxHub's expertise in patient identification and delivering drug benefit information to the physician at the point of care complements SureScripts' focus on electronic prescription routing from the physician's office to the pharmacy. The merger combines these strengths with a shared focus on more access to patient medication history to form a single suite of comprehensive services. The new organization will enable physicians to securely access vital health information when caring for their patients through a fast and efficient health information exchange. This will allow them to transmit electronic prescriptions and renewal requests to both retail and mail-order pharmacies.

More information regarding SureScripts and RxHub is discussed in Chapters 6, 7, 8, and 9.

In late June 2008, the Drug Enforcement Administration published proposed regulations that would allow for electronic prescribing of controlled substances.[2] The public comment for these regulations will run until September 25, 2008. In effect, these regulations would allow eligible prescribers with controlled substance prescriptive authority to transmit prescriptions electronically to pharmacies. As it is currently written, these proposed regulations will require physicians to register with law-enforcement agencies and allow routine audits of prescription records.[3] On a weekly basis, pharmacists will be required to verify the licensure and "good standing" of the prescribers transmitting such prescriptions.[3] In addition, if electronic systems were to be breached by hackers or others, the DEA must be notified by the pharmacy within 24 hours.[3] The ramifications of e-prescribing of controlled substances affecting patients, physicians and pharmacists is discussed in detail in Chapters 5, 6, 8, and 9.

These recent developments will not be isolated in their occurrence. As e-prescribing gains more and more of a foothold in the delivery of health care services, many more changes and impacts will occur with regular frequency.

References

1. SureScripts. *Retail Pharmacies and Largest Pharmacy Benefit Managers Announce Merger of e-Prescribing Networks—Improving Safety, Accuracy, Efficiency of Prescription Medicines for Patients Nationwide.* Available at: http://www.surescripts.com/pressrelease-detail.aspx?id=137&ptype=surescripts. Accessed July 23, 2008.
2. U.S. Department of Justice, Drug Enforcement Administration. *DEA Issues Proposed Regulations to Allow Electronic Prescriptions for Controlled Substances* [June 27, 2008]. Available at: http://www.usdoj.gov/dea/pubs/pressrel/pr062708.html. Accessed July 24, 2008.
3. DoBias M. Docs liable under DEA's proposed e-regulations. *Mod Healthcare.* July 11, 2008;Online. Available at: http://www.modernhealthcare.com/apps/pbcs.dll/article?AID=/20080711/REG/771055892/1029/FREE. Accessed July 24, 2008.

ONE

e-Prescribing: What It Is and Why It Is a Sea Change for Delivery of Medical Care

Introduction

The manner in which physicians have ordered medications for patients has remained the same for over a century. Now, new technologies are revolutionizing how prescriptions are processed. Information technology (IT) has impacted much of what we do in all facets of our lives. New technologies are now dramatically influencing health care providers. These technologies make the handwritten prescription seem like an archaic link to the past. Introducing and accepting change in any profession has always been a challenge; this is certainly the case in the practice of medicine. The advent of computerization has brought new technologies into play for many facets of our health seeking, including our health care access and utilization. Please note that electronic prescribing and attendant components have spun off a new series of acronyms. The Glossary at the end of this book contains most, if not all, the acronyms we will explore and provides a brief definition of each.

What is *electronic prescribing* (also known as e-prescribing)? It has been defined as the use of computing devices to enter, modify, review, and output or communicate drug prescriptions.[1] The earliest application of physicians ordering medications and other therapies via computer was in hospitals in the 1970s. Now, the use of e-prescribing in the health care delivery system is expanding rapidly.

Prior to this emerging technology for transmitting medication orders, physicians placed orders by hand for well over a century in virtually the same manner. They wrote orders for drugs on a piece of paper (prescription blanks are at present 4.25 × 5.5 inches) with the only difference being whether the printing on the blank was portrait or landscape in presentation. Prescriptions have also been transmitted from physician to pharmacies via oral orders sent by telephone or via facsimile transmission.

What Has Been the Impetus for e-Prescribing?

Why is there a need to change how drugs are ordered by physicians? One of the earliest mentions of e-prescribing in medical literature was in the early 1990s; the study profiled use of computers for various tasks, including refill prescription prescribing (repeat prescribing). A small percentage of the Welsh physicians in this study (11%) used computers for this purpose.[2] The authors concluded the paper with this exhortation: "Mechanisms to encourage greater and more sophisticated use of computers and information technology need to be explored."[2(p.94)] In the United States in the mid-1990s, electronic prescriptions were touted as a means to more accurately transmit physicians' orders.[3] Elsewhere, authors have suggested that e-prescribing will lead to enhanced medication use in hospitals and beyond.[4] Is e-prescribing a case in which, because the technology is available to be used, it must in fact be used?

Rate of Adoption

In August 2007, Alaska became the last of the 50 states to enable e-prescribing. Varying estimates have suggested that 21% of physicians have access to IT-accessible e-prescribing.[5] A recent article noted that although a vast majority of physicians surveyed (85%) support e-prescribing (thinking it is a "good idea"), only 7% actually use the technology at present.[6,7]

The Problems with Paper Prescriptions

There have been calls for a decrease in frank errors of commission that occur in the prescribing of medications. These errors of commission due to illegible handwriting on the part of physicians, errors in reading prescriptions on the part of pharmacists, or errors of pharmacy technicians that were not subsequently caught by the supervising pharmacist have led to an uncalculated degree of morbidity and mortality. There is simply not a mechanism to catch and collate such errors on a widespread basis.[8] Regardless of who is to blame, transcribing prescriptions from one hand to another can be fraught with errors.

Figure 1-1 provides a listing of the major causes of death in the United States. Note the line indicating the number of deaths due to adverse medical events, which is estimated to be between 44,000 and 98,000.[9] This may be an understated value; in many cases a drug-related error leading to a death will not be listed as a cause of death for a patient. However, one of the factors posited to lead to this value is the illegibility of physicians' handwriting.

FIGURE 1-1 **Leading Causes of Death and Adverse Medical Events Resulting in Death, 2005**

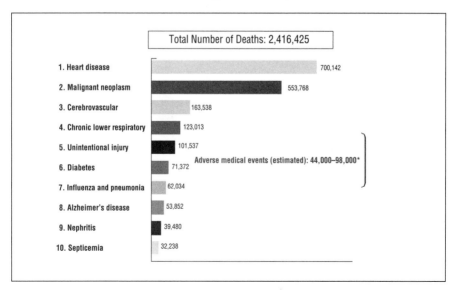

Other problems with prescription writing include the altering of prescriptions by patients seeking additional drugs, patients writing the prescriptions themselves on stolen prescription blanks, or other gaps in the system of writing and dispensing medications. Effective October 1, 2007, prescriptions transmitted for patients in the Medicaid programs throughout the United States are now required to be written on a tamper-resistant prescription blank. The following is about the Centers for Medicare and Medicaid Services (CMS) directive on this issue:[10]

- As of October 1, 2007, in order for outpatient drugs to be reimbursable by Medicaid, all written, nonelectronic prescriptions must be executed on tamper-resistant pads.

- CMS has outlined 3 baseline characteristics of tamper-resistant prescription pads, but each state will define which features it will require to meet those characteristics in order to be considered tamper-resistant. To be considered tamper resistant, on October 1, 2007, a prescription pad must have at least one of the following 3 characteristics:[10]
  - One or more industry-recognized features designed to prevent unauthorized copying of a completed or blank prescription form;
  - One or more industry-recognized features designed to prevent the erasure or modification of information written on the prescription by the prescriber;
  - One or more industry-recognized features designed to prevent the use of counterfeit prescription forms.

- States will require that the prescription pad have all 3 characteristics no later than October 1, 2008, to be considered tamper-resistant.

- Several states have laws and regulations concerning mandatory, tamper-resistant prescription pad programs, which were in effect prior to the passage of section 7002(b). CMS deems that the tamper-resistant prescription pad characteristics required by these states' laws and regulations meet or exceed the baseline standard, as set forth above.

- Each state must decide whether they will accept prescriptions written in another state with different tamper-proof standards.

- CMS believes that both e-prescribing and use of tamper-resistant prescription pads will reduce the number of unauthorized, improperly altered, and counterfeit prescriptions.

- The new requirement does not apply when the prescription is electronic, faxed, or verbal. (CMS encourages the use of e-prescribing).

- Other means of prescribing on an emergency basis is allowed provided that a prescriber provides a verbal, faxed, electronic, or compliant prescription within 72 hours after the date on which the prescription is filled.

Thus, e-prescribing has been codified into practices through the clout of CMS and the specter of nonpayment of claims if the guidance is not followed.

e-Prescribing as a Solution

Programs to transmit physician orders electronically that are in place in hospital settings have been advocated for use in outpatient settings as well. Adubofour and colleagues have noted:[11(p.1562)]

> Medication errors are being closely scrutinized as part of these hospital-based efforts. Most Americans, however, receive their healthcare in the ambulatory primary care setting. Primary care physicians are involved in the writing of several million prescriptions annually. The steps underway in our hospitals to reduce medication errors should occur concurrently with steps to increase awareness of this problem in the out-patient setting.

e-Prescribing has been suggested as a remedy for many of the prescription prescribing and dispensing ills that are present in the U.S. health care delivery system. e-Prescribing will more easily take care of many of the errors that tamper-resistant prescription blanks are meant to address.[12] By using secure and hacker-resistant transmission of prescriptions, less effort will be needed to ease the current problem of tampering with traditional paper prescription blanks.

The end result of e-prescribing may be a dramatic difference in how prescription writing occurs, but the means to reach this goal will be challenging.[13] The process of change will certainly not be an easy transition.[14] Not the least of the important issues that need to be addressed is who will ultimately be responsible for funding the transition and maintenance of meshing systems.[15] However, when this transition is finally accomplished, patients and providers alike will reap the rewards of changing to an e-prescribing environment.[16] One suggestion for speeding up the transition to e-prescribing is to provide incentives to providers.[17,18]

So, if the process has been implemented in numerous patient care settings in the health care delivery system and seems to provide rewards for patients and providers alike, why does this book need to be written?

Impediments to Adoption

In December 2007, Congress passed legislation that reauthorized Medicare, Medicaid, and State Children's Health Insurance Programs (SCHIP) without an IT mandate requested by the Bush administration.[19] This rebuff to strong lobbying efforts by personnel from the Bush administration is indicative of the problems that remain before widespread adoption takes place.

e-Prescribing will be a major shift in how prescriptions are transmitted from physicians' offices to pharmacies, and hundreds of thousands of physicians' offices will need to be electronically equipped to transfer prescriptions. Newly graduated doctors may be more facile with this technology and its application; however, older physicians will need information, elaboration, and descriptors of what this new technology is all about.

Physicians have lagged behind other professions in utilizing electronic communication. Studies have shown that only 25% of physicians communicate with their patients via email.[20] This percentage will increase as electronic medical records (EMR), health information technology (health IT), and governmental influences become more commonplace and accepted by the medical community.

Health profession practitioners, health profession students in training, IT practitioners, and those who propose e-prescribing and deal indirectly with the outcomes of e-prescribing (such as third-party prescription drug plans and governmental agencies like CMS)—in total, hundreds of thousands of practitioners—will be affected. Parallel interest areas will develop within the pharmaceutical manufacturing and distribution system. In addition, health administrators dealing with clinic administration and group practices will be involved in e-prescribing, not as prescription prescribers but as implementers, enablers, and/or facilitators.

One issue that needs to be explored and amplified is the general feeling that e-prescribing will solve many drug-related errors in prescribing and transcribing. As with any computer program, appropriate care will need to be taken when training physicians on how to use them. e-Prescribing in and of itself will not solve all drug-related error issues.

There also have been suggestions that e-prescribing will enhance patient compliance with medications. e-Prescribing has been in place for a while in countries that have national health insurance schemes and programs, and data from European studies do not necessarily bear out this.[21] This new technology will be effective only as far as it directly improves patient care and patient outcomes and does so in an economically sound fashion.

Summary

e-Prescribing will no doubt transform the practice of medicine and related professions. However, multiple aspects of this new technology need to be addressed, including the economic effects, the social/political ramifications, the effects upon professions and professional collaborations, and most importantly, the influence of e-prescribing on patients and patient care.

References

1. Teich JM, Marchibroda JM. *Electronic Prescribing: Toward Maximum Value and Rapid Adoption* (A Report of the Electronic Prescribing Initiative). Washington, DC: eHealth Initiative; April 14, 2004.
2. Goves JR, Davies T, Reilly T. Computerisation of primary care in Wales. *Br Med J.* 1991; 303(6794):93–94.
3. Siwicki B. Electronic prescriptions: just what the doctor ordered. *Health Data Manag.* 1995;3(10):62–68.
4. Schiff GD, Rucker TD. Computerized prescribing: building the electronic infrastructure for better medication usage. *JAMA.* 1998;280(6):516–517.
5. Grossman JM, Gerland A, Reed MC, Fahlman C. Physicians' experiences using commercial e-prescribing systems. *Health Aff.* 2007;Web exclusive:w393–w404.
6. Pharmacy Times News Brief. Small percentage of MDs use e-prescribing. *Pharm Times.* December 2006. Available at: http://www.pharmacytimes.com/issues/articles/2006-12_4145.asp. Accessed June 3, 2008.
7. Glendinning D. Pharmacy benefit managers push Medicare e-prescribing. *Amer Med News.* August 13, 2007. Available at: http://www.ama-assn.org/amednews/2007/08/13/gvsd0813.htm#s1. Accessed August 17, 2007.
8. Agency for Healthcare Research and Quality. *2007 National Healthcare Quality Report* (AHRQ Pub. No. 08-0040). Rockville, MD: U.S. Department of Health and Human Services, Agency for Healthcare Research and Quality; 2008.
9. Kohn L, Corrigan J, Donaldson M. *To Err Is Human: Building a Safer Health System.* Washington, DC: Institute of Medicine, National Academy Press; 1999.

10. Smith DG. Letter to state Medicaid director. August 17, 2007. Available at: http://www.cms.hhs.gov/SMDL/downloads/SMD081707.pdf. Accessed May 27, 2008.

11. Adubofour KO, Keenan CR, Daftary A, et al. Strategies to reduce medication errors in ambulatory practice. *J Natl Med Assoc*. 2004;96(12):1558–1564.

12. Bertola D. Pads are first step toward eliminating forgeries. *Business First of Buffalo*. August 24, 2007. Available at: http://www.bizjournals.com/buffalo/stories/2007/08/27/focus4.html?b=1188187200%5e1510189. Accessed May 27, 2008.

13. Ridinger MH. The electronic prescription conundrum: why "e-Rx" isn't so "e-Z." *Clin Pharmacol Ther*. 2007;81(1):13–15.

14. Bergeron B. Medication errors and e-prescribing: solutions and limitations. *J Med Pract Manage*. 2004;20(3):152–153.

15. Thomas N, Fifer SK. The combination of collaborative drug therapy management and e-prescribing. *Manage Care Interf*. 2003;16(1):38–42,46.

16. Sternberg DJ. Make life a little easier. Online prescriptions reap rewards for doctors and patients. *Mark Health Serv*. 2003;23(2):44–46.

17. Ochs J. e-Prescribing gets more enticing. *Manage Care*. 2002;11(2):60–61.

18. Mellin A. e-Prescribing: an opportunity for process re-engineering. *Health Manag Tech*. 2002;23(1):42,44,47.

19. HDM Breaking News. I.T. mandate out of Medicare bill. *Health Data Manag*. December 21, 2007. Available at: http://www.healthdatamanagement.com/news/mandate_legislation_Medicare25383-1.html. Accessed May 27, 2008.

20. Liebhaber A, Grossman JM. Physicians slow to adopt patient e-mail (Data Bulletin No. 32). *Center for Studying Health System Change*. September 2006. Available at: http://www.hschange.org/CONTENT/875. Accessed May 27, 2008.

21. Kansanaho H, Puumalainen I, Varunki M, Ahonen R, Airaksinen M. Implementation of a professional program in Finnish community pharmacies in 2000–2002. *Pat Educ Couns*. 2005;57(3):272–279.

TWO

Introduction to Electronic Media and Influences on Health and Medical Care

Introduction

Electronic media have a variety of influences on physicians and many other health professionals. Governmental (e.g., state, federal), organizational (e.g., American Medical Association, American Medical Informatics Association), and other interested parties all have promoted electronic media adoption and utilization in the health care system.

According to the U.S. Department of Health and Human Services (HHS), health IT is a pervasive opportunity for many agencies that lie within the HHS purview. The HHS health IT Web site (http://www.hhs.gov/healthit) provides the rationale, background, current and future efforts in progress or to be implemented and descriptions of how health IT can help transform the practice of medicine and delivery of health care and enable more accurate assessments of the outcomes of care.

Descriptors on the HHS health IT Web site suggest that health IT will allow for:[1]

comprehensive management of medical information and its secure exchange between health care consumers and providers. Further, the broad and implemented use of health IT will:

- Improve health care quality;
- Prevent medical errors;
- Reduce health care costs;
- Increase administrative efficiencies;
- Decrease paperwork; and
- Expand access to affordable care.

In addition, interoperable health IT will improve individual patient care, but it will also bring many public health benefits including:

- Early detection of infectious disease outbreaks around the country;
- Improved tracking of chronic disease management; and
- Evaluation of health care based on value enabled by the collection of de-identified price and quality information that can be compared.

Federal Efforts in the Early 21st Century

An important component of President Bush's health IT plans was the e-prescribing regulation proposed by the CMS within the Department of HHS. This e-prescribing regulation sought to improve the care seniors receive in Medicare by helping to bring electronic prescriptions to seniors when the prescription drug benefit took effect in January 2006.[2] Another goal was to stimulate broader adoption of e-prescribing across the entire health care system. When President Bush signed into law the Medicare Prescription Drug, Improvement, and Modernization Act of 2003, a component of the bill called for standards to enable e-prescribing for the Medicare Part D program with a full roll-out by 2009.[3] (Please see Appendix A for a copy of the federal mandate for instituting e-prescribing.) It was thought that e-prescribing would improve the quality and safety of patient care through reduced medication errors and the monitoring for adverse drug reactions and could increase efficiency in physician offices.

As a connector between patients, doctors, and pharmacies accelerated adoption of e-prescribing in Medicare was thought to help spur e-prescribing and the adoption of electronic health records throughout the nation's health care system. (Please see Appendix B for a 21st-century time line for the implementation of e-prescribing.)

The Initiative to Update America's Health Care System

According to information related to health IT on the White House Web site:[4]

> . . . information technology is changing American industry. At the end of the 1990s, most American industries were spending approximately $8,000 per worker for IT, but the health care industry was investing only approximately $1,000 per worker. The United States has always been innovative with medical care, but continues to face major hurdles in our health information systems as we move into the 21st century. Despite spending over $1.6 trillion on health care as a Nation, there are still serious concerns about high costs, avoidable medical errors, administrative inefficiencies, and poor coordination—all of which are closely connected to the failure to incorporate health information technology into our health care system.
>
> Current health information systems use an outdated, paper-based system: The innovation that has made our medical care the world's best has not been applied to our health information systems. America's medical professionals are the best and brightest in the world, and set the standard for the world. President Bush is working to ensure that America's health information systems match the high quality of the Nation's medical personnel.

The following materials are from the public domain Web site of the White House, from a page entitled *Fact Sheet: Improving Care and Saving Lives Through Health IT.*[4]

> America's patients deserve an up-to-date medical information system. A patient's vital medical information is scattered, and full records are often

unavailable at the time of care, and especially during emergency care. Patients lack access to useful, credible health information to choose the best treatment for their needs, and manage their own wellness. America's doctors should have a high-quality, health information system to best serve their patients. Physicians are not able to keep vast amounts of information about drugs, interactions, and guidelines easily at hand to select the best treatments for their patients. Medical orders and prescriptions must be handwritten and are too often misunderstood.

President Bush's Plan to Improve Care and Save Lives Through Health IT: President Bush's Health Information Technology Plan is continuing to address the longstanding problems in the Nation's health care system. The President believes that better health information technology is essential to improve America's health care system, and he is committed to his goal of assuring that most Americans have electronic health records within the next 10 years. Electronic health records will share information privately and securely among and between health care providers when authorized by the patient.

To achieve his 10-year goal, the President has taken the following steps to promote coordinated public- and private-sector efforts that will accelerate broader adoption of health care information technology:

Using the Federal Government to Foster Greater Adoption of Health Information Technology: Bush wanted to develop plans to build on progress already made in this area by fostering regional collaborations and demonstration projects that will test the effectiveness of Health IT and encourage widespread adoption. Bush also directed the Federal government to coordinate its health information systems so that care delivered by the Federal government, reimbursement, and oversight is more efficient and cost-effective.

Adopting Uniform Health Information Standards to Allow Medical Information to Be Stored and Easily Shared Electronically While Maintaining Privacy: Over the last several years, HHS has been collaborating with the private sector and other Federal agencies to identify and endorse voluntary standards necessary for health information to be shared safely and securely among health care providers. The results of these projects include standards for transmitting X-rays over the Internet; electronic lab results transmitted to physicians for immediate analysis, diagnosis and treatment—assuring a prompt response and eliminating errors and duplicative testing due to lost laboratory reports; and standardized electronic prescriptions, which save time for patients and help to avoid serious medical errors.

The New National Health Information Technology Coordinator is providing national leadership and the coordination necessary to achieve the President's 10-year goal. Dr. David Brailer, former Senior Fellow at the Health Technology Center in San Francisco, is guiding ongoing work on health information standards and processes to identify and implement the various steps needed to support and encourage health information technology in the public and private health care delivery systems. Dr. Brailer is also coordinating partnerships between government agencies and private sector stakeholders to speed the adoption of health information technology.

Computerized Physician Order Entry

More than 10 years ago, Bates wrote about the continuing problem of medication errors in hospitals and pointed to several strategies to help improve the problem, including computerized physician order entry (CPOE).[5]

The Leapfrog Group

General Motors Corp, IBM, AT&T, General Electric, Boeing, and 91 other employers collaborated in 2001 to form the Leapfrog Group so as to leap forward with work to increase health care quality in the United States. According to information provided by the Leapfrog Group on its Web site:[6(p.2)]

> In 1998 a group of large employers came together to discuss how they could work together to use the way they purchased health care to have an influence on its quality and affordability. They recognized that there was a dysfunction in the health care market place. Employers were spending billions of dollars on health care for their employees with no way of assessing its quality or comparing health care providers. Funding to set up Leapfrog came from the Business Roundtable (BRT), and The Leapfrog Group was officially launched in November 2000.

The Leapfrog Group uses the term "leap" to signify significant improvement actions that have been implemented. For example, the group's leaps adhere to four primary criteria:

1. There is overwhelming scientific evidence that these quality and safety leaps will significantly reduce preventable medical mistakes.
2. Their implementation by the health industry is feasible in the near term.
3. Consumers can readily appreciate their value.
4. Health plans, purchasers, or consumers can easily ascertain their presence or absence in selecting among health care providers.

These leaps are a practical first step in using purchasing power to improve hospital safety and quality.

Standards Implemented by the Leapfrog Group
The Leapfrog Group has worked to develop standards and guiding principles for implementation of health IT on a broad scale in the United States.[7] Leapfrog's CPOE standard requires hospitals to:[6(p.2)]

- Assure that physicians enter at least 75% of medication orders via a computer system that includes prescribing-error prevention software.
- Demonstrate that their inpatient CPOE system can alert physicians of at least 50% of common, serious prescribing errors, using a testing protocol now under development by First Consulting Group and the Institute for Safe Medication Practices (this criterion for the Leap will not count towards the hospital's publicly reported status on this Leap until the test is available).
- Require that physicians electronically document a reason for overriding an interception prior to doing so.

According to the Leapfrog Group, CPOE systems are "electronic prescribing systems that intercept errors when they most commonly occur—at the time medications are ordered. With CPOE, physicians enter orders into a computer rather than on paper. Orders are integrated with patient information, including laboratory and prescription data."[6(p.1)] After the entry of preliminary data the physician's order is electronically checked for errors or other problems. The Leapfrog Group indicates that CPOE benefits include:[6(p.1)]

- Prompts that warn against the possibility of drug interaction, allergy, or overdose
- Accurate, current information that helps physicians keep up with new drugs as they are introduced into the market
- Drug-specific information that eliminates confusion among drug names that sound alike
- Improved communication between physicians and pharmacists
- Reduced health care costs due to improved efficiencies

Other CPOE Advocates

Others have studied CPOE and its potential and actual utility in improving health care.[8] Kuperman and Gibson note, "the costs of CPOE are substantial both in terms of technology and organizational process analysis and redesign, system implementation, and user training and support."[8(p.31)] They also point out, however, that there are substantial quality problems throughout the health care system and that information technology such as CPOE is a promising technology that allows physicians to enter orders into a computer instead of handwriting them. Because orders are electronically entered and data detected, Kuperman and Gibson[8] posit that CPOE can substantially decrease the overuse, underuse, and misuse of health care services.[8] They go on to state that studies have documented that CPOE can decrease costs, shorten length of stay, decrease medical errors, and improve compliance with several types of guidelines.[8]

CPOE in Medicine, Nursing, and Pharmacy

Other applications of CPOE with subpopulations have been reported in the literature of medicine, nursing, and pharmacy. Medication errors were shown to decrease in a retrospective cohort study with a pediatric hospital population, thus avoiding injuries that would have resulted because of medication errors.[9] The nursing literature also contains articles detailing the positive attributes of CPOE and suggests the technology can be the next step in the prevention of medication errors.[10] The influence of CPOE has a global reach as well. CPOE has been implemented in Europe with intended positive results occurring as projected.[11]

In a study evaluating the impact of CPOE and team intervention (several specific process changes that included changing the role of pharmacists) on the incidence of serious medication errors, researchers found that there was a 55% decrease in serious medication errors.[12] This study concluded that the team intervention produced no additional benefit over CPOE alone.[12] In spite of the potential and documented benefits of CPOE, however, less than 5% of hospitals in the United States currently have CPOE in place and require it to be used by attending or staff physicians.[12]

Bar Coding and Its Applications

Bar coding can be defined as the use of a linear bar code on a label or other strip that contains a series of optically readable lines that are a unique identifier. The modern bar code era began in the late 1940s, and its first application was in the food/grocery industry. Bar coding allowed for increased accuracy in the scanning and pricing of consumer goods. Applications of bar coding have been implemented elsewhere, including health and health care.

The Utility of Bar Coding

Bar coding initially was implemented in hospitals as a mechanism to control inventory (drugs, central supplies, surgical instruments, intravenous admixtures, etc). The application of bar coding to decrease medication administration errors has been a very positive application of the technology.[14] Success has been tangible in numerous health care systems incorporating bar coding technology.[15] Bar coding has also been used in Canada and Europe with similar stories of successful outcomes.[16]

Schulmeister notes, "safety experts currently recommend using technology to prevent medication errors. CPOE, automated medication-dispensing machines, and bar coding are a few of the technologies being advocated to promote safety with chemotherapy regimens."[17(p.201)] As expected, bar-code medication administration systems can prevent medication errors; however, health care organizations must be aware of identified failure points in bar coding that may contribute to errors.[18] Nothing in health care should be considered a fail-safe solution, including bar coding.[18]

Bar Coding as One Part of a Systems Approach

Using bar coding as but one part of a systems approach to dealing with care and care delivery has been advocated.[19] Crane and Crane note that "medication errors in hospital settings are considered both widespread and costly to the American healthcare system; yet, it is tractable to available solutions."[20(p.3)] They suggest a solution consisting of "a systems approach—failure mode effects analysis (FMEA)—in combination with emerging technologies, such as a decision support system (DSS) with integrated real-time medical informatics, electronic medical records (EMR), computer physician order entry (CPOE), bar coding, automated dispensing machines (ADM), and robotics."[20(p.8)] Perrin and Simpson note, "medication administration recording and supply management are complex and interrelated processes. The integration of bar codes and radio frequency identification tags are viewed as critical in achieving effective and safe patient care."[21(p.33)] They also call for alignment and integration of the varying systems for optimal success. Careful planning is called for to optimally achieve the desired outcomes.[21]

Proposals have been made to reduce the frequency of errors with medication use. In a white paper extolling information technology as a means to decrease medical errors, Bates and colleagues lay out specific recommendations such as, "to implement provider order entry systems, especially computerized prescribing; to implement bar-coding for medications, blood, devices, and patients; and to utilize modern electronic systems to communicate key pieces of asynchronous data such as markedly abnormal laboratory values."[22(p.399)]

Governmental Actions

For over a decade, the U.S. Food and Drug Administration (FDA) has required bar coding for use with blood products and drugs to enhance safety.[23] Other government health care entities have implemented bar coding as one part of a systems approach to enhancement of quality. The Veterans Health Administration (VHA) has implemented nationally mandated initiatives including "bar coding of all medications and use of computerized medical records that include order entry, laboratory and imaging results, and all encounter notes."[24]

Not a Cure-All

Human frailties and mistakes make no system foolproof. Bar coding of patients with wristbands only works if the correct patient is given the correct wristband. Horror stories have been related when mistakes such as this are made.[25] As previously mentioned, a combination of technologies shows the most promise.[26]

Clinical Decision Support Systems

Numerous calls and attempts have been made to apply evidence to health care. Computerized norms through clinical decision support systems (CDSS) have emerged as sophisticated tools to bring evidence into the practices of health care practitioners. In *Crossing the Quality Chasm: A New Health System for the 21st Century*, it is suggested that "far more sophisticated clinical decision support systems will be needed to assist clinicians and patients in selecting the best treatment options and delivering safe and effective care."[27] The authors go on to assert: "Certain types of clinical decision support applications most notably preventive service reminder systems and drug dosing systems have been demonstrated to improve clinical decisions and should be adopted on a widespread basis."[27]

The integration of technologies, including CDSS, on medication errors throughout the medication-use process has shown positive effects: "Most prescribing errors decreased significantly in the categories monitored, specifically drug allergy detection, excessive dosing, and incomplete or unclear orders."[28(p.1969)] CDSS alerts were shown to "improve therapeutic drug monitoring in patients with renal insufficiency and in patients receiving drugs with narrow therapeutic ranges."[28(p.1973)]

Health IT, including CPOE with CDSS, has been proposed as an important systems-based approach for reducing medication errors and preventable drug-related injuries. Subramanian and colleagues note that physicians and long-term care (LTC) facilities will bear the brunt of payment for these systems.[29] With this being the case, physicians and LTC facilities will need to be incentivized to use these technologies.[29]

Other health professions have entered the world of CDSS. In a study of 15 databases, Randell et al found that CDSS had an inconsistent effect on nursing performance and patient outcomes.[30] Interactions with CDSS are complex, so care is urged in evaluating the overall effectiveness of CDSS.[30]

CDSS has found applications in numerous settings, such as in public health emergencies.[31] With the need to act quickly and uniformly, this might be a perfect application for CDSS. In a study examining physician preferences for types of CDSS, "data showed that physicians prefer to use certain handheld CDS tools in clinical settings."[32] In a study of CDSS for chronic health failure, "barriers to implementation included relatively low computer skills among family physicians and a lack of complexity within CDSS in addressing the wider nonmedical needs of patients."[33(p.504)] The authors suggest that "improving computer skills, and integrating CDSS into referral pathways and requests for investigation may be ways of enhancing the use of this technology."[33(p.504)]

As was the case with bar coding, CDSS has been implemented elsewhere in the world. A Dutch study using CDSS combined with a nurse practitioner indicated that diabetic patients fared better with the combined CDSS and nurse practitioner as opposed to physician care.[34]

Summary

As noted in this chapter, there are many technologies available to enable more accurate diagnosis, treatment, and transmission of orders, laboratory values, and record keeping. A concerted and integrated approach seems to be the most advantageous path to follow.

References

1. Department of Health and Human Services. *Health Information Technology Home*. Available at: http://www.hhs.gov/healthit. Accessed May 26, 2008.
2. Centers for Medicare and Medicaid Studies. *Summary of H.R. 1: Medicare Prescription Drug, Improvement, and Modernization Act of 2003* (Public Law 108-173). April 2004. Available at: http://www.cms.hhs.gov/MMAUpdate/downloads/PL108-173summary.pdf. Accessed May 27, 2008.
3. Department of Health and Human Services, Centers for Medicare and Medicaid Services. Standards for e-prescribing under Medicare Part D and identification of backward compatible version of adopted standard for e-prescribing and the Medicare Prescriptions Drug Program (Version 8.1). *Fed Reg*. April 7, 2008;73(67):18917. Available at: http://www.federalregistersearch.com/2008/4/7/08-1094.asp. Accessed May 29, 2008.
4. The White House, Office of the Press Secretary. *Fact Sheet: Improving Care and Saving Lives Through Health IT*. Available at: http://www.whitehouse.gov/news/releases/2005/01/20050127-2.html. Accessed May 29, 2008.

5. Bates DW. Medication errors: how common are they and what can be done to prevent them? *Drug Saf.* 1996;15:303–310.

6. The LeapfrogGroup. *Factsheet: Computer Physician Order Entry.* April 24, 2008 (Revision). Available at: http://www.leapfroggroup.org/media/file/Leapfrog-Computer_Physician_Order_Entry_Fact_Sheet.pdf. Accessed May 27, 2008.

7. The LeapfrogGoup. *The LeapfrogGroup Factsheet.* March 2008. Available at: http://www.leapfroggroup.org/media/file/The_Leapfrog_Group_Fact_Sheet_03_2008.pdf. Accessed May 26, 2008.

8. Kuperman GJ, Gibson RF. Computer physician order entry: benefits, costs, and issues. *Ann Intern Med.* 2003;139(1):31–39.

9. King WJ, Paice N, Rangrej J, Forestell GJ, Swartz R. The effect of computerized physician order entry on medication errors and adverse drug events in pediatric inpatients. *Pediatr.* 2003;112(3):506–509.

10. Jech O. Next step in preventing med errors. *RN.* 2001;64:46–49.

11. Arend A. The CPOE system in Luxembourg. *Eur J Hosp Pharm Sci.* 2006;12(3);52–53.

12. Bates DW, Leape LL, Cullen DJ, et al. Effect of computerized physician order entry and a team intervention on prevention of serious medication errors. *JAMA.* 1998;280;1311–1316.

13. Mekhijan HS, Kumar RR, Kuehn L, Bentley TD, Teater P, Thomas A, Payne B, Ahmad A. Immediate benefits realized following implementation of physician order entry at an academic medical center. *J Am Med Inform Assoc.* 2002; 9(5):529–539.

14. Kester M. Bar coding at the bedside: New England hospital implements an automated point-of-care medication administration system to reduce medication errors and their associated complications. *Health Manag Technol.* 2004;25(5):42–44.

15. Tribble DA. Bar coding a must for patient safety. *Am J Health Syst Pharm.* 2002;59(7): 667–668.

16. Holmes L. A survey of bar coding in Canadian teaching hospitals. *Dimens Health Serv.* 1987;64:23–25.

17. Schulmeister L. Ten simple strategies to prevent chemotherapy errors. *Clin J Oncol Nurs.* 2005;9(2):201–205.

18. Cochran GL, Jones KJ, Brockman J, Skinner A, Hicks RW. Errors prevented by and associated with bar-code medication administration systems. *Jt Comm J Qual Patient Saf.* 2007;33(5):293–301.

19. Wright AA, Katz IT. Bar coding for patient safety. *N Engl J Med.* 2005;353(15):1640.

20. Crane J, Crane FG. Preventing medication errors in hospitals through a systems approach and technological innovation: a prescription for 2010. *Hosp Top.* 2006;84(4):3–8.

21. Perrin RA, Simpson N. RFID and bar codes—critical importance in enhancing safe patient care. *J Healthc Inf Manag.* 2004;18(4):33–39.

22. Bates DW, Cohen M, Leape LL, Overhage JM, Shabot MM, Sheridan T. Reducing the frequency of errors in medicine using information technology. *J Am Med Inform Assoc.* 2001;8(4):398–399.

23. Association of Schools of Public Health. Medication bar coding and safety reporting to improve patient safety. *Public Health Rep.* 2003;118(3):75.

24. Weeks WB, Bagian JP. Developing a culture of safety in the Veterans Health Administration. *Eff Clin Pract.* 2000;3(6):270–276.

25. McDonald CJ. Computerization can create safety hazards: a bar-coding near miss. *Ann Intern Med.* 2006;144(7):510–516.

26. Hagland M. Safe ways. Hospitals looking to improve patient safety are turning to CPOE, bar coding and e-prescribing. *Healthc Inform.* 2004;21(8):20–25.

27. Committee on Quality of Health Care in America, Institute of Medicine. *Crossing the Quality Chasm: A New Health System in the 21st Century.* Washington, DC: National Academy of Sciences, Institute of Medicine; 2001. Available at: http://www.nap.edu/catalog/10027.html. Accessed October 18, 2007.

28. Mahoney CD, Berard-Collins CM, Coleman R, Amaral JF, Cotter CM. Effects of an integrated clinical information system on medication safety in a multi-hospital setting. *Am J Health Syst Pharm.* 2007;64(18):1969–1977.

29. Subramanian S, Hoover S, Gilman B, Field TS, Mutter R, Gurwitz JH. Computerized physician order entry with clinical decision support in long-term care facilities: costs and benefits to stakeholders. *J Am Geriatr Soc.* 2007;55(9):1451–1457.

30. Randell R, Mitchell N, Dowding D, Cullum N, Thompson C. Effects of computerized decision support systems on nursing performance and patient outcomes: a systematic review. *J Health Serv Res Policy.* 2007;12(4):242–251.

31. McGowan JJ, Richwine MW, Overhage JM. A sustainable, multi-organizational model for decision support during public health emergencies. *Stud Health Technol Inform.* 2007; 129:1465–1466.

32. Yu F Jr, Houston TK, Ray MN, Garner DQ, Berner ES. Patterns of use of handheld clinical decision support tools in the clinical setting. *Med Decis Making.* 2007;27(6):744–753. Available at: doi:10.1177/0272989X07305321.

33. Leslie SJ, Denvir MA. Clinical decision support software for chronic heart failure. *Crit Pathw Cardiol.* 2007;6(3):121–126.

34. Cleveringa FG, Gorter KJ, van den Donk M, Pijman PL, Rutten GE. Task delegation and computerized decision support reduce coronary heart disease risk factors in type 2 diabetes patients in primary care. *Diabetes Technol Ther.* 2007;9(5):473–481.

THREE

e-Prescribing: What Is It and What Is It All About?

Introduction

Various U.S. federal government agencies, varying state agencies, and private entities have all impacted the emergence and acceptance of e-prescribing. Some of these impacts have been via legislative fiat, and some via state rules and regulations pertaining to pharmacy and medical practice within a state. Each, in different ways, from legislation to regulation to enabling software to financing third-party programs, have converged to hasten the entry of e-prescribing into the mainstream health care system in the United States.

Federal Government Involvement in e-Prescribing

As noted in Chapter 1, e-prescribing refers to the transfer of prescription orders electronically from a prescriber to a pharmacy with ultimate delivery to patients or patient representatives. e-Prescribing also enables pharmacies to access refill records electronically and proceed with prescription processing without the need to contact physicians' offices. In effect, facsimile transmission of prescription orders has been done electronically, but e-prescribing details a level of interactivity between prescriber and pharmacy that is different.

Bell et al define e-prescribing as:[1(p.60)]

Electronic prescribing (e-prescribing), which we define as clinicians' computerized ordering of specific medication regimens for individual patients, offers the potential to substantially reduce medication errors and also to improve health care efficiency.

CMS describes e-prescribing as follows:[2]

e-Prescribing—a prescriber's ability to electronically send an accurate, error-free and understandable prescription directly to a pharmacy from the point-of-care—is an important element in improving the quality of patient care. The inclusion of electronic prescribing in the Medicare Modernization Act (MMA) of 2003 gave momentum to the movement, and the July 2006 Institute of Medicine report on the role of e-prescribing in reducing medication errors has received widespread publicity, helping to build awareness of e-prescribing's role in enhancing patient safety. Developing the standards that will facilitate e-prescribing is one of the key action items in the governments plan to expedite the adoption of electronic medical records and build a national electronic health information infrastructure in the United States.

CMS is heavily involved in promoting e-prescribing as a cost saving, error reduction, and streamlining component to Medicare and Medicaid programs in the United States.

Other Governmental Agencies and Regulations Pertaining to e-Prescribing

Online ordering of many commodities is commonplace at present; this process of prescription flow through the system in this fashion is very new to health care and health care delivery. Also, this process for health and health care is more regulated than other "commodities." Prescription orders are regulated by:

- State medical boards
- State pharmacy boards

- Federal agencies
  - ○ Food and Drug Administration
  - ○ Drug Enforcement Administration
- Funding agencies
  - ○ Centers for Medicare and Medicaid Services
    - • Medicare
    - • Medicaid
- Individual states
  - ○ Joint financing of Medicaid with the federal government

Why Is e-Prescribing So Different?

Please see **Figure 3-1** for a schematic drawing of the traditional method of transference of prescriptions from prescriber to pharmacist to delivery to patient or patient representative. In this traditional method, prescribers can be allopathic physicians (MDs), osteopathic physicians (DOs), dentists, podiatrists, nurse practitioners, physician assistants, and optometrists (ODs). As noted on the diagram, pharmacy benefit management companies (PBMs) and/or insurers may operate a mail order pharmacy and receive prescriptions from prescribers; then they dispense the medications directly to the patient. This pathway from doctor to patient has—as was previously noted—changed little from the long-term to the recent past. With the exception of the addition of telephoned and faxed prescription orders, this pathway has remained unchanged for decades.

FIGURE 3-1 **Traditional Method of the Transfer of Prescriptions**

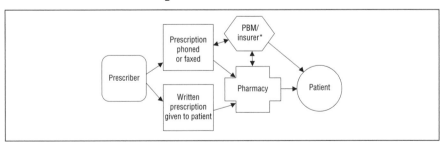

*The arrow from *PBM/insurer* to *Patient* reflects the situation where a pharmacy benefit management company (PBM) operates a mail order pharmacy that provides prescriptions to patients.

Figure 3-2 depicts how e-prescribing changes this dynamic. The various governmental regulatory controls over prescribing are still in play with e-prescribing; it is just the underlying dynamic processes that are dramatically different. The time saving and error avoiding aspects of e-prescribing are benefits that will be explored in later chapters. But, these tangible benefits are significant and will dramatically alter how prescribing, dispensing, and providing prescriptions will change in the near and long-term future. In Figure 3-2, the double directed red arrow from electronic device to PBM/insurer circumvents the traditional option of filling prescriptions in local pharmacies. The green arrow indicates the interplay between PBM/insurers and pharmacies are still a possibility. But, these systems have been set up so that PBM/insurers with mail order pharmacies are directly hardwired into this process and do in fact lead to avoidance of using the traditional pharmacy for prescription processing. This will not always happen, but the possibilities and capabilities are such that this scenario is much more likely to happen than not in most cases.

RxHub

The RxHub Patient Health Information Network™ is the only network in the United States providing authorized physicians with secure access at the point of

FIGURE 3-2   **The e-Prescribing Transfer of Prescriptions**

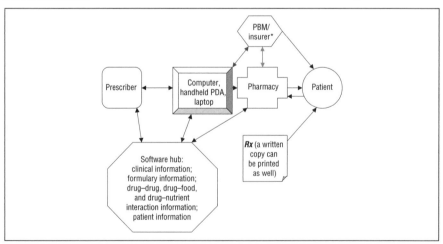

*The arrow from *PBM/insurer* to *Patient* reflects the situation where a pharmacy benefit management company (PBM) operates a mail order pharmacy that provides prescriptions to patients.

care to prescription eligibility, formulary and benefits, and medication history information (for consenting patients).[3] This real-time, decision-support information is used by physicians to effectively manage a patient's use of medications, and it enables the most clinically appropriate and cost-effective medication therapy to be prescribed. The flow of information and subsequent prescriptions through the RxHub system is presented in **Figure 3-3**.

FIGURE 3-3 **What Is RxHub Informed e-Prescribing?**

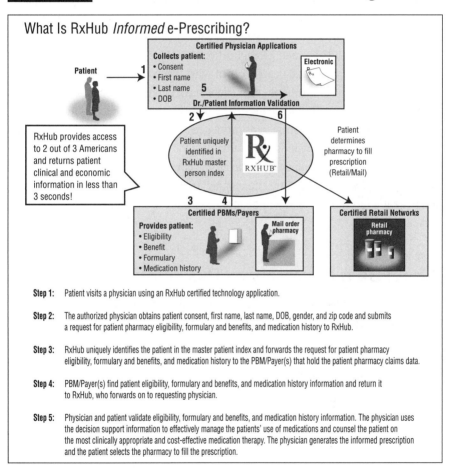

What Is RxHub *Informed* e-Prescribing?

Step 1: Patient visits a physician using an RxHub certified technology application.

Step 2: The authorized physician obtains patient consent, first name, last name, DOB, gender, and zip code and submits a request for patient pharmacy eligibility, formulary and benefits, and medication history to RxHub.

Step 3: RxHub uniquely identifies the patient in the master patient index and forwards the request for patient pharmacy eligibility, formulary and benefits, and medication history to the PBM/Payer(s) that hold the patient pharmacy claims data.

Step 4: PBM/Payer(s) find patient eligibility, formulary and benefits, and medication history information and return it to RxHub, who forwards on to requesting physician.

Step 5: Physician and patient validate eligibility, formulary and benefits, and medication history information. The physician uses the decision support information to effectively manage the patients' use of medications and counsel the patient on the most clinically appropriate and cost-effective medication therapy. The physician generates the informed prescription and the patient selects the pharmacy to fill the prescription.

Source: RxHub National Patient Health Information Network. *RxHub FAQ.* Available at: http://www.rxhub.net/images/pdf/RxHub_FAQ.pdf. Accessed June 9, 2008. Reprinted with permission of RxHub.

Some Current Issues

e-Prescribing accounts for roughly 5% to 7% of physicians' prescriptions at present.[4] Due to impending CMS requirements set to be finalized and implemented by 2009, e-prescribing of prescriptions for 39 million Medicare Part D clients will be firmly established.[2] In fact, Medicare is suggesting reimbursing roughly $12,000 for every office where outpatient prescriptions are to be written by physicians.[5] This total amount for all physicians in office-based practices or group practices will exceed $400 million.[5] With thousands of physicians' offices to be electronically equipped to transfer prescriptions, a major shift in how prescriptions are transmitted from physicians' offices to pharmacies will take place. Newly graduated doctors may be more facile with this technology and its application; however, older physicians will need information, elaboration, and descriptors of what this new technology is all about.

As noted earlier in this book, physicians have lagged behind other professions in utilizing electronic communication. The percentage of adopters will increase as EMRs, health IT, and governmental influences become more commonplace and accepted by the medical community. Certainly, other health professionals with varying degrees of acceptance and use of electronic communication technology, such as pharmacists, physician assistants, nurse practitioners, managed care organizations, and patient advocacy groups, will be affected by the emerging e-prescribing wave approaching.

What Else Is Necessary at This Point?

According to a CMS report to Congress, several changes are necessary for optimum and full operability of e-prescribing.[2] This report notes:[2(p.23–24)]

> The Structured and Codified SIG standard needs additional work with reference to field definitions and examples, field naming conventions, and clarifications of field use where new codes are recommended, such as the SIG Free Text Indicator field. It is imperative that the prescriber's instructions be translated exactly into e-prescribing and pharmacy practice management systems to reduce medication errors, decrease healthcare costs and improve patient safety. For example, contradictions with other structured fields exist, and there are limitations on directions for topical drugs (such as the area of application). The PRN designation (pro

re nata or "as needed") could be interpreted as either "as needed" or "as required", and the standard does not allow for quick revisions for new drug administration. Mistranslations and contradictions in dosage/timing directions leave room for misinterpretation and error. With additional development, the standard may provide a controlled vocabulary that reflects prescriber thinking, offers structure and simplicity, and improves communications between prescribers and pharmacies. Analysis shows that the standard is not technically able to support this function for use in Medicare Part D e-prescribing in its current state.

Government Involvement in e-Prescribing via Medicare Part D

One of the key considerations of the widespread adoption of e-prescribing will revolve around third-party requirements for prescription submissions for payment. When the Medicare Prescription Drug, Improvement, and Modernization Act of 2003 (Public Law 108-173) enabled the provision of a new voluntary prescription drug benefit under Medicare, an impetus for adoption of e-prescribing became apparent. Although e-prescribing will be optional for physicians and pharmacies, Medicare will require drug plans participating in the new prescription benefit to support electronic prescribing.[6] Because of this, e-prescribing will be commonplace and accepted more as years progress and more enrollees obtain outpatient prescription coverage and subsequent use of prescription medications.

A 2007 CMS report to Congress described the results of CMS-funded pilot projects serving as an impetus for further adoption of e-prescribing, These pilot projects noted that e-prescribing can be more widely adopted and can serve to benefit patients and providers alike through a streamlined drug prescribing and prescription acquisition process. The report states:[2]

> On November 7, 2005, CMS published foundation standards that became effective on January 1, 2006. These standards apply to all electronic prescribing done under Part D of the MMA. The foundation standards cover:
>
> - Transactions between prescribers (who write prescriptions) and dispensers (who fill prescriptions) for new prescriptions; refill

requests and responses; prescription change requests and responses; prescription cancellation, request, and response; and related messaging and administrative transactions;

- Eligibility and benefits queries and responses between prescribers and Part D sponsors;
- Eligibility queries between dispensers and Part D sponsors.

MMA required CMS to implement pilot projects to test additional standards. These additional standards were pilot tested in 2006. They are:

- Formulary and benefit information
- Prior authorization requirements
- Medication history requirements
- Structured and codified dosing information (e.g., the SIG)
- RxNorm

The results of the pilot test were announced in a report to Congress in April 2007 and were the basis for an NPRM proposing additional standards that was published on November 16, 2007.

What Is "RxNorm"?

RxNorm is a term for the process of normalizing information components of prescription medications. The unified medical language system provided by the U.S. National Library of Medicine from the National Institutes of Health and the Department of Health and Human Services describes RxNorm as follows:[7]

RxNorm provides standard names for clinical drugs (active ingredient plus the strength of the drug plus various dosage forms) and for dosage forms as administered to patients. RxNorm provides links from clinical drugs, both branded and generic, to their active ingredients, drug components (active ingredient plus strength), and related brand names (for multisource products). National Drug Codes (NDCs) for specific drug products (where there are often many NDCs for a single product) are linked to that product in RxNorm. RxNorm links its names to many of the drug vocabularies commonly used in pharmacy management and drug interaction software, including those of First Databank, Micromedex, Medi-Span, Gold Standard Alchemy, and Multum. By providing links between these vocabularies, RxNorm can mediate messages between systems not using the same software and vocabulary.

RxNorm is one of a suite of designated standards for use in U.S. Federal Government systems for the electronic exchange of clinical health information.

Remaining Questions and Summary

In a Government Accountability Office (GAO) report in January 2007, the GAO recommended that HHS:[4]

- Define and implement an overall privacy approach that identifies milestones for integrating the outcomes of its initiatives
- Ensure that key privacy principles are fully addressed
- Address challenges associated with the nationwide exchange of health information

So, key questions remain regarding the implementation of e-prescribing. Who will pay for its implementation?[9] How will data be shared?[10] Will there be exclusivity factors involved with proprietary treatment of data and processes?[11] Concerns about the privacy of personal health information are not new![12] Please see Appendix C for a compilation of the various federal laws and regulations that are set in place to protect personal health information.

References

1. Bell DS, Cretin S, Marken RS, Landman AB. A conceptual framework for evaluating outpatient electronic prescribing systems based on their functional capabilities. *J Amer Med Inform Assoc*. 2004;11:60–70. Available at: doi:10.1197/jamia.M1374.
2. Leavitt MO. *Pilot Testing of Initial Electronic Prescribing Standards—Cooperative Agreements Required Under Section 1860D-(4) (e) of the Social Security Act as Amended by the Medicare Prescription Drug, Improvement, and Modernization Action (MMA) of 2003*. Available at: http://www.cms.hhs.gov/EPrescribing. Accessed November 24, 2007.

3. RxHub National Patient Health Information Network. *Frequently Asked Questions*. Available at: http://www.rxhub.net/index.php?option=com_content&task=view&id=40&Itemid=53. Accessed June 6, 2008.
4. Teich JM, Marchibroda JM. Recommendations for optimal design and implementation to improve care, increase efficiency and reduce costs in ambulatory care. In: *Electronic Prescribing: Toward Maximum Value and Rapid Adoption* (A Report of the Electronic Prescribing Initiative). Washington, DC: eHealth Initiative; April 14, 2004.
5. Rosenfeld R, Bernasek C, Mendelson D. Medicare's next voyage: encouraging physicians to adopt health information technology. *Health Aff*. 2005;24(5):1138–1146.
6. Centers for Medicare and Medicaid Studies. *e-Prescribing Overview*. Available at: http://www.cms.hhs.gov/EPrescribing. Accessed May 28, 2008.
7. U.S. National Library of Medicine, National Institutes of Health. *Unified Medical Language System*. Available at: http://www.nlm.nih.gov/research/umls/rxnorm. Accessed May 29, 2008.
8. Koontz LD, Powner DA. *Health Information Technology. Early Efforts Initiated, but Comprehensive Privacy Approach Needed for National Strategy* (GAO-07-238). Washington, DC: U.S. Government Accountability Office; February 2007. Available at: http://www.gao.gov/new.items/d07400t.pdf. Accessed May 28, 2008.
9. Douglas S, Bell DS, Friedman MA. e-Prescribing and the Medicare Modernization Act of 2003. *Health Aff*. 2005;24(5):1159–1169.
10. Gottlieb LK, Stone EM, Stone D, Dunbrack LA, Calladine J. Regulatory and policy barriers to effective clinical data exchange: lessons learned from MedsInfo-ED. *Health Aff*. 2005;24(5):1197–1204.
11. Hammond WE. The making and adoption of health data standards. *Health Aff*. 2005;24(5):1205–1213.
12. Gavison R. Privacy and the limits of law. *Yale L J*. 1980;89(3):421–471.

CHAPTER

FOUR

The Enduring Experiential and Strategic Underpinning of e-Prescribing

Introduction

Successful e-prescribing systems are dependent upon technology sufficiency, interoperability, and security of information to be accessed and that which is to be provided. The technology must be such that numerous physicians can access a site simultaneously with ease of transmission and realize appropriate access as necessary. Security of the information transmitted and accessed is of paramount concern and must be the starting point for any e-prescribing system.

Historically, IT has been a component of health care delivery. In 1962, the Illinois Department of Health used an IBM 1401 computer to manage public health and maternal and child health data and to communicate disease control.[1] (This computer was 5 feet tall by 3 feet wide and had a storage capacity of 16 Kilobytes [KB]—for comparative purposes, 1024 KB = 1 Megabyte [MB]!)

Traditional Method of Prescription Writing Versus e-Prescribing

A schematic representation of the traditional method for transfer of prescriptions from physician to pharmacist and dispensing to patients the finished product is presented in **Figure 4-1**. As previously noted, this process for writing prescriptions, dispensing medications, and furnishing the finished product to patients has remained virtually the same for decades. The only innovations may have been telephone or facsimile transfer of prescriptions from physicians to pharmacists. Certainly, the impact of PBMs and/or insurers has been ubiquitous in the recent past as far as being a financial gatekeeper impacting pharmacists, physicians, and—most importantly—patients. PBMs monitor formularies, prescribing limits (30 days supply or more), payments to pharmacies, and co-payments required of patients before given access to medications.

e-Prescribing

e-Prescribing offers a technologically advanced option for order transfer from physician to pharmacist and subsequent processing of the prescription(s) for patient use. Please see **Figure 4-2** for a schematic representation of how e-prescribing can be implemented.

FIGURE 4-1   **Traditional Method of the Transfer of Prescriptions**

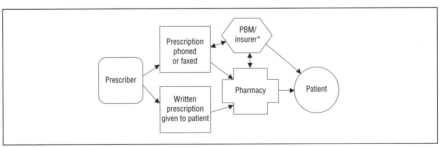

*The arrow from *PBM/insurer* to *Patient* reflects the situation where a pharmacy benefit management company (PBM) operates a mail order pharmacy that provides prescriptions to patients.

FIGURE 4.2   **The e-Prescribing Transfer of Prescriptions**

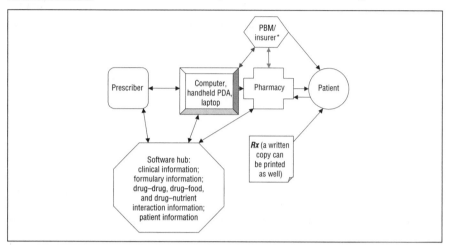

*The arrow from *PBM/insurer* to *Patient* reflects the situation where a pharmacy benefit management company (PBM) operates a mail order pharmacy that provides prescriptions to patients.

Interoperability

Interoperability requirements are necessary so that the interface of CPOE, computerized patient records (CPR), and decision making aids can be accomplished with differing systems that maintain the same standards for use for different points of access.[2] There are numerous vendors of computer-based technologies in the health care environment, and each tries to ensure customer loyalty by designing systems that do not interface with competing systems.[3] This competition leads to fragmentation with numerous products and clinical decision aids, limited interoperability, a need for regular and often expensive technical support, and increased costs.

In order to realize the full benefits of interoperable medical information networks, health care data needs to be standardized, and these uniform sets of technical standards related to medical procedures, billing, reimbursement, administrative, and other practice issues will be widely available and accessible nationwide.[4] Standardization will help to eliminate the silo approach to access and control of computerized patient information. The U.S. Veterans

Administration health IT system, known as VISTA, is a successful example of how a medical information network can interface between pharmacy, laboratory, and other clinical systems and subsystems.[5]

For utility to occur, different applications must allow for communication efficiency between remote telemedicine, telerobotic devices that can interface with CPOE, CPR, and electronic clinical decision aids in health care system environments. Efficiency in delivery and access to information will lead to increases in health care quality indices.[6]

Security of Information

The enabling legislation for application of e-prescribing technology is explicit in its description of safeguards necessary for e-prescribing implementation.[7] The CMS legislation provides:[7]

> The new e-prescribing standards should be designed to enable transmission of basic prescription data to and from doctors and pharmacists, as well as information about the patient's drug utilization history, possible drug interactions, the drug plan (including information about the formulary and cost-sharing), and information about lower-cost therapeutically appropriate alternatives. The standards must comply with HIPAA privacy rules. Messaging unrelated to appropriate prescribing (such as marketing) will not be allowed.

For any system to be acceptable, guarantees of security of data received and transmitted must be a basic tenet for use.

Experiential

The need to protect personal health information expands as does the application of health information and need for exchange of information. A breach in security—placing individuals at risk for leakage of health information—for systems that gather and control large amounts of data is a threat that will not diminish in the future and with future applications of technology.

Strategic Opportunities with e-Prescribing

According to the Joint Commission, "Eliminating handwriting in health care altogether is the preferred solution to illegible handwriting, and many believe that technology will provide the means to fulfilling this solution. In the short term, organizations can focus on improving handwriting, but there must be a long-term solution aimed at communicating electronically."[8](p.3)

Federal Laws Impacting e-Prescribing

Numerous laws enacted at the federal level have been guiding efforts to ensure the privacy of health information.[9] Please see **Table 4-1** for a listing of the titles of these laws. A more complete descriptor of these federal laws can be found in Appendix C. The complexity of the concept of maintaining the privacy of personal health information is reflected in the sheer number of these laws and the continuing

TABLE 4-1   **Various U.S. Federal Laws Protecting Patient Rights to Confidentiality**

HIPAA
Privacy Act of 1974
Freedom of Information Act of 1966
Social Security Act
Veterans Omnibus Health Care Act of 1976
Medicare Prescription Drug, Improvement, and Modernization Act of 2003
Clinical Laboratory Improvement Amendments of 1988
Public Health Service Act Health Omnibus Programs Extension of 1988
Public Health Service Act Federal Confidentiality Requirements for Substance Abuse Patient
    Records
Family Educational Rights and Privacy Act; Protection of Pupil Rights Amendment
Americans with Disabilities Act
Financial Modernization (Gramm-Leach-Bliley) Act of 1999

Adapted from: Koontz LD, Powner DA. *Health Information Technology. Early Efforts Initiated, but Comprehensive Privacy Approach Needed for National Strategy* (GAO-07-238). Washington, DC: U.S. Government Accountability Office; February 2007. Available at: http://www.gao.gov/new.items/d07400t.pdf. Accessed June 5, 2008.

enactment of laws on a regular basis that fill in the gap of security of personal health information. Strategically, the MMA of 2003 has the most significant impact upon the security of health information as it pertains to e-prescribing.[9]

The Medicare Prescription Drug, Improvement, and Modernization Act of 2003

The federal law that really initiated much of the activity concerning e-prescribing was the Medicare Prescription Drug, Improvement, and Modernization Act of 2003. Selected segments of this law are detailed in Appendix D. These selected segments are most pertinent to e-prescribing and its effects on medicine and pharmacy.

Basic Requirements

A series of tables (**Table 4-2**, **Table 4-3**, and **Table 4-4**) list data points necessary for e-prescribing accuracy, system requirements, and handheld device requirements to enable e-prescribing. These listings should not be considered a definitive listing for each category, but they do indicate what is necessary for e-prescribing systems. Regarding the listings in Table 4-2, it should be noted that for cautionary advice provided for a drug, a drug interaction, a contraindicated drug, or a drug allergy indicator, there would be override capabilities. This means the prescriber can proceed with a prescribed entry even if the system is indicating that the drug should not be prescribed for various reasons. These types of "gates" have been in place for years in pharmacy computer systems but have always had the capability of a warning being overridden.

CMS Pilot Testing of e-Prescribing

In November 2007, the CMS released the following information regarding e-prescribing and regulatory requirements.[10] These sections that follow are reprinted from the monograph *Pilot Testing of Initial Electronic Prescribing Standards–Cooperative Agreements Required Under Section 1860D-(4) (e) of the Social Security Act as Amended by the Medicare Prescription Drug, Improvement, and Modernization Act (MMA) of 2003*.[10] This document is in the public domain.

TABLE 4-2	**Required Data Points Ideal for e-Prescribing Accuracy**

- Activity reports: patient specific information
- Allergy data: drugs and other agents
- Available drug listing: for prescribing drugs
  - Formularies, specific for patient availability
- Drug reactions and interactions
  - Drug/allergy interactions
  - Drug/drug interactions
  - Drug/food interactions
  - Drug/herbal supplement interactions
- Drug reference
- Drug reports: patient medication history
- Eligibility check: insurance eligibility
- Favorite prescription list
  - For the prescribing physician, the most commonly prescribed drugs specific to the physician
- Generic medication listing
- Global pharmacy list: all pharmacies eligible to be used
  - Mail-order pharmacy
- Last office visit
- Medication history download for each patient
- Patient medication history
- Practice pharmacy list: favorite of physician or patient
- Patient schedule
- Patient sharing: other physicians seeing patient can be viewed
- Patient demographics: age, gender, other pertinent notations
- Pharmacy search: area specific or accessible at a specific point in time
- Prescription report: all drugs the physician(s) has prescribed
- Rapid medication entry
  - A character recognition system that displays the drugs with these letters that have been typed
- Renewals/refills: available for each of the patient's prescriptions
- Referrals: from and to the physician entering the data
- User preferences: favorite dosing parameters that are physician specific can be added

TABLE 4-3 **Representative System Requirements for e-Prescribing**

A Windows compatible personal computer (PC)

Required computer memory: 64 MB of RAM (128 MB for Windows 2000, more for Windows XP or Windows Vista)

Available hard disk space: 20 MB

Processor speed: 200 mHz

Browser: Internet Explorer 5.0 or higher with cipher strength of 128-bit encryption or Netscape 4.7 or higher with cipher strength of 128-bit encryption

Internet connection (DSL or faster is recommended, dial-up may not be reasonable)

Printer is not required; useful if hard copy of prescriptions is desired by the patient

Computer monitor (any will suffice)

Software loaded on the computer to enable e-prescribing activities to be conducted

TABLE 4-4 **Considerations for Handheld Computers (PDAs)**

Access to a device specific software application and subsequent downloading of the software to the device, e.g., a Palm Pilot, Blackberry, or Dell device, wireless access or bluetooth technology

A USB, serial port, or 802.11b (WIFI) for the PDA (whichever the PDA uses for HotSync or ActiveSync)

4 MB free hard disk space

Palm

Appropriate operating system, e.g., Palm OS 3.5 or higher or other operating system

Memory: 16 MB of total memory with at least 5 MB available

Pocket PC

Operating system: Windows 2003 Mobile, Pocket PC 2003, and Windows Mobile 5.0

Memory: 8 MB available

Other devices by differing manufacturers will need to be tested by the sponsoring provider of software for ascertaining compatibility

Section 101 of the Medicare Prescription Drug, Improvement, and Modernization Act of 2003 (MMA) (Pub. L. 108-173) amended Title XVIII of the Social Security Act (the Act) to establish the Voluntary Prescription Drug Benefit Program. Included in the provisions of section 1860D-4(e) of the Act is the requirement that the electronic transmission of prescriptions and certain other information for covered Part D drugs prescribed for Part D eligible individuals comply with standards adopted by the Secretary.

Medicare Prescription Drug Plan (PDP) sponsors, Medicare Advantage (MA) organizations offering Medicare Advantage-Prescription Drug Plans (MA-PD) and other Part D sponsors are required to support and comply with electronic prescribing standards once they are in effect, including any standards that were in effect when the drug benefit began in 2006.

[Author's Note: The following section is interesting to me in that there is a descriptor of the "voluntary" aspects of e-prescribing uptake and subsequent use. In this author's view, these voluntary allowances may be in place, but one will not be able to practice and benefit in the future without the uptake of e-prescribing into practices.]

There is no requirement that providers or pharmacies implement e-prescribing. However, providers and pharmacies that electronically transmit prescription and certain other information for covered drugs prescribed for Medicare Part D eligible beneficiaries are required to comply with any applicable final standards that are in effect.

The MMA requires the adoption of final standards to support the e-prescribing program described in the MMA. The MMA mandates e-prescribing standards that allow for information exchange, to the extent feasible, on an interactive, real-time basis; and allow for the exchange of information only as it relates to the appropriate prescribing of drugs, including quality assurance measures and systems. The MMA requires that standards for e-prescribing be consistent with the objectives of improving patient safety, quality of care, and efficiencies.

The MMA requires standards for conveying:

1. Eligibility and benefits information, including the drugs included in the applicable formulary, and tiered formulary structure, and any requirements for prior authorization.
2. The following information with respect to the prescribing and dispensing of a covered Part D drug:

    a. information on the drug being prescribed or dispensed and other drugs listed on the medication history, including information on drug-drug interactions, warning or cautions, and when indicated, dosage adjustments; and

   b. information on the availability of lower cost, therapeutically appropriate alternatives (if any) for the drug prescribed.

3. Information that relates to the medical history concerning an individual and related to a covered Part D drug being prescribed or dispensed, upon request of the professional or pharmacist involved.

In addition, the MMA requires design criteria for these standards so that they are compatible with general health information technology standards, permit electronic exchange of drug labeling and drug listing information maintained by the Food and Drug Administration (FDA) and the National Library of Medicine (NLM), and, to the extent practicable, they do not impose an undue administrative burden on the industry.

To provide for efficient implementation of the requirements, section 1860D-4(e) of the Act required the Secretary to conduct a pilot project to test initial standards recognized under section 1860D-4(e)(4)(A) of the Act, prior to issuing the final standards in accordance with section 1860D-4(e)(4)(D) of the Act, and provide a report to the Congress by April 1, 2007, on his evaluation of the pilot project. Section 1860D-4(e)(4)(C)(ii) of the Act allows for an exception to the requirement to pilot test initial standards if, after consultation with standards setting organizations (SSOs) and industry users, the Secretary has determined that there already is adequate industry experience for a standard. Any such "foundation standards" can be proposed and adopted through notice and comment rulemaking as final standards without pilot testing.

Section 1860D-4(e) of the Act also requires that the Secretary promulgate final uniform standards by no later than April 1, 2008.

[Author's Note: The document continues with a description of e-prescribing standards and the relationship with the National Committee on Vital and Health Statistics.]

The MMA charged the National Committee on Vital and Health Statistics (NCVHS) with developing, in consultation with various named parties, recommendations for uniform standards that would enable electronic prescribing in ambulatory care settings, and promote patient safety and quality health care. The NCVHS held hearings to obtain testimony regarding which standards were needed to support e-prescribing; how MMA requirements were supported or not supported by current standards (i.e., standards gaps and limitations); and any related issues that might affect e-prescribing implementation or acceptance.

Standards are the essential building blocks for the widespread adoption of electronic prescribing and other health information technologies (HIT). The standards that have been recognized for e-prescribing under the MMA are published specifications that were developed and/or approved by standard setting organizations (SSOs). These standards establish common vocabulary, content, technical or other specific criteria that serve as a rule, a guideline, or a definition that would promote interoperability amongst users. This concept of "interoperability" entails various systems successfully inter-communicating with one another through standard mechanisms (i.e., "standard transactions") that convey standardized content (i.e., common data elements and vocabularies). Such standards, combined with a real time and secure network, would ensure that providers have instant, secure access to accurate and timely patient information through an electronic health record or similar application. The result would be the ability to coordinate and monitor patient care across different providers. Collecting and transmitting patient data is a complex process. The data elements and transmission specifications must "match" at both the source and destination computer systems, which is only achievable with adherence to the same standards.

From expert testimony, the NCVHS determined that standards needed to be identified for basic prescribing functions between a prescriber and pharmacy; to support eligibility verifications (including individual formularies); and for decision support functionality (e.g., drug utilization review functions), while identifying standards gaps and limitations in all of these instances. The NCVHS identified three types of e-prescribing standards as necessary to support electronic prescribing. They are: message format standards that provide communication protocols and data content requirements (including those that support medication decision making); terminologies to ensure data comparability and interoperability; and unique identifiers for all relevant entities within

the e-prescribing process. The NCVHS held hearings and industry participants debated the criteria for immediate adoption as well as whether specific standards should be recommended as foundation standards. That
recommended criteria included that the standard was from a standard setting organization that was accredited by the American National Standards
Institute (ANSI); that the standard generally has been implemented by entities to which the final standard will be applied in multiple e-prescribing
programs with more than one external health care partner; and that the standard is recognized by key industry stakeholders as the industry standard.
Three standards met these criteria and were recommended by the NCVHS
for adoption as foundation standards for the new Part D requirement.

[Author's Note: The National Council for Prescription Drug Programs (NCPDP)
began in 1977 and—now with 1,500 members representing various segments of
pharmacy—has been crucially important for the maturing of the third-party prescription drug scene in the United States. Without the work of NCPDP, the sub-
mission and payment of drug claims at the current degree of success would not be
possible.]

Regulatory Requirements: After reviewing the NCVHS recommendations, the Secretary concurred with NCVHS' conclusion that the three
standards recommended as having had adequate industry experience could
in fact be adopted as final standards through notice and comment rulemaking without pilot testing. These standards were called "foundation"
standards, because while they do not support the full range of e-prescribing functionality, they are a base onto which other standards can be built.
   The proposed foundation standards were:

- The NCPDP Telecommunications Standard Version 5, Release 1
  and the NCPDP Batch.
- Standard Batch Implementation Guide Version 1.1 for eligibility
  communications between retail pharmacy dispensers and Part D
  sponsors.
- The Accredited Standards Committee (ASC) X12N 270/271 Version 4010 and Addenda to Version 4010 for eligibility communications between prescribers and Part D sponsors.

- The NCPDP SCRIPT Standard Version 5, Release 0 for exchanging new prescriptions, changes, renewals, cancellations and certain other transactions between prescribers and dispensers.

- Formulary representation and medication history standards, if certain conditions were met and the identified standards had adequate industry experience.

Public comments supported adoption of the first three standards, and HHS published a final rule on November 7, 2005 (70 FR 67568) adopting them, effective January 1, 2006, when the Part D benefit took effect. This rule also established a streamlined process for updating adopted standards by identifying backward compatible, later versions of the standards that were not also HIPAA standards. Use of such subsequent versions of an adopted standard would be voluntary. Subsequent industry input indicated that the adopted SCRIPT standard, Version 5.0, should be updated with a later version of the standard (Version 8, Release 1). Using the streamlined process, HHS published an Interim Final Rule on June 23, 2006 (71 FR 36020) updating the adopted SCRIPT standard, thereby permitting either version to be used.

While e-prescribing is voluntary under the Medicare prescription drug benefit, providers and pharmacies that transmit prescriptions for Medicare covered drugs electronically are required to comply with any applicable final standards that are in effect. Further, all Part D plans are required to maintain e-prescribing systems that conform to the final standards.

Summary

The technology necessary to successfully implement e-prescribing on a large scale is in place and ready for broad implementation. What is now necessary are a series of important components:

- Physician acceptance of the technology
- Increased physician realization of the importance for medicine to accept a computer literate approach to health and health care

- A firm grasp of the costs and necessary enablers to fully implement e-prescribing

- Pharmacy acceptance of e-prescribing on a large scale

- A better grasp than is currently available to ascertain who will absorb the costs of e-prescribing

- A concerted effort toward interoperability

- Safeguards to ensure safety of data entry and access for interested parties

- An approach to health IT that encompasses e-prescribing as but one component of the necessary steps to fully implement all that health IT has to offer health care and health care delivery

- An avoidance of sequestering this technology into a silo mentality

References

1. Lumpkin JR, Richards MS. Transforming the public health information infrastructure. *Health Aff.* 2002;21(6):45–56.

2. Brailer DJ. Translating ideals for health information technology into practice. *Health Aff.* May 25, 2004;Web exclusive:w318–w320. Available at: doi:10.1377/hlthaff.w4.318.

3. Poon EG, Blumenthal D, Jaggi T, et al [My paper]. Overcoming barriers to adopting and implementing computerized physician order entry systems in U.S. hospitals. *Health Aff.* 2004;23(4):184–190.

4. Hammond WE. The role of standards in electronic prescribing. *Health Aff.* May 25, 2004;Web exclusive:w325. Available at: doi:10.1377/hlthaff.W4.325.

5. Chaffee BW, Bonasso J. Strategies for pharmacy integration and pharmacy information system interfaces. Part 1: History and pharmacy integration options. *Am J Health Syst Pharm.* 2004;61:602–606.

6. Brailer DJ. Interoperability: the key to future health care system. *Health Aff.* January 19, 2005;Web exclusive:w19–w25. Available at: doi:10.1377/hlthaff.w5.19.

7. Centers for Medicare and Medicaid Studies. *Summary of H.R. 1: Medicare Prescription Drug, Improvement, and Modernization Act of 2003* (Pub L No. 108-173). Available at: http://www.cms.hhs.gov/MMAUpdate/downloads/PL108-173summary.pdf. Accessed June 5, 2008.

8. Joint Commission on Accreditation of Healthcare Organizations. Even legible handwriting can cause harm: moving toward electronic communications. *Jt Comm Perspect Patient Saf.* 2006:6(12):3–4.

9. Koontz LD, Powner DA. *Health Information Technology. Early Efforts Initiated, but Comprehensive Privacy Approach Needed for National Strategy* (GAO-07-2007).

Washington, DC: U.S. Government Accountability Office; February 2007. Available at: http://www.gao.gov/new.items/d07400t.pdf. Accessed May 28, 2008.

10. Leavitt MO. *Pilot Testing of Initial Electronic Prescribing Standards—Cooperative Agreements Required Under Section 1860D-(4) (e) of the Social Security Act as Amended by the Medicare Prescription Drug, Improvement, and Modernization Act (MMA) of 2003*. Available at: http://www.cms.hhs.gov/EPrescribing. Accessed November 24, 2007.

FIVE

The Benefits of e-Prescribing

Introduction

Some of the benefits of e-prescribing have been alluded to in earlier chapters. In this chapter, more specific information about the advantages offered by e-prescribing will be presented. The potential realized benefits assigned to e-prescribing are dependent upon physician acceptance of the changes inherent in e-prescribing. The e-prescribing movement has gained momentum, and it is instructive to examine how the technology has been adopted as rapidly as it has been.

Why Is e-Prescribing Seen as So Important?

According to the Institute of Medicine, preventable medication errors are estimated to be responsible for more than 1.5 million injuries and 7,000 deaths each year in the United States.[1] Dealing with the morbidity associated with medication errors costs billions extra to provide follow-up care for those affected. CMS estimates that if e-prescribing would be adopted by physicians in Medicare at a level of 18%, for a 5-year period, cost savings would amount to $4 billion, and an estimated 3 million adverse drug events could be avoided.[2] Thus, we can see why e-prescribing has been promoted as a benefit for the Medicare and Medicaid programs.

Calls for e-Prescribing Implementation

There have been calls for a rapid implementation of e-prescribing from many different sources. Entrepreneurial, therapeutically driven, politically motivated, and quality of care enhancement efforts have merged motives into a perfect storm that has pushed the e-prescribing momentum further along than might be expected at this juncture.

Quality of Care and Political Intersections

From quality of care standpoints, musings by Newt Gingrich and John Kerry have focused many individuals' attentions upon e-prescribing. Although an unlikely pair of discussants, Gingrich and Kerry have called on the U.S. government to improve the quality of health care by addressing the issue of preventable medication errors.[2] Gingrich and Kerry support the adoption of e-prescribing and explain its benefits. The pair also recommends ways in which the government can persuade doctors to adopt e-prescribing. They suggest: "One reason for this mess is that 95% of prescriptions are transmitted using 5,000-year-old technology: pen and paper."[2(p.A20)]

Gingrich and Kerry further suggest:[2(p.A20)]

> The benefits are clear and compelling. When a doctor "writes" an electronic prescription, a computer can warn of potentially dangerous interactions with other medications or allergies and thereby prevent thousands of unnecessary hospitalizations each year. e-Prescribing can also let a physician know whether a drug is covered by a patient's insurance or whether an alternative generic is available at a fraction of the cost. One initiative led by Chrysler, General Motors and Ford to encourage doctors to write e-prescriptions in the Detroit region has generated more than one million prescription alerts that have saved lives and money.

Kerry and Gingrich argue that e-prescribing should be a requirement of doing business with Medicare for physicians.

Public-Private Efforts

The American Health Information Community (AHIC) is a federal advisory body with public and private membership chartered in 2005 to make recommendations to the Secretary of HHS on how to accelerate the development and adoption of health IT. AHIC was formed by the secretary of HHS to help advance efforts to achieve President Bush's goal for most Americans to have access to secure electronic health records by 2014. On November 28, 2007, AHIC recommended that HHS Secretary Mike Leavitt seek authority from Congress to mandate e-prescribing in Medicare.[3] This has spurred activity to examine how e-prescribing can be instituted expeditiously.

Entrepreneurial Support for e-Prescribing

In 2004, a new coalition of software vendors formed an advocacy group for e-prescribing initiatives. Their efforts had an economic focus, but it offered a perspective that needs to be considered as well. The coalition, Cafe Rx, sought to "tackle the thorny problems of practice change, industry collaboration and medication politics that could keep the e-prescription movement stalled long after initial questions of standards adoption are resolved."[4(p.14)] Realizing that fewer than 5% of the nation's doctors were prescribing electronically, the groups sought to promote the benefits of e-prescribing.[4]

Institute Systems in Outpatient Settings Similar to Institutional Systems

Calls have been made for implementation of systems linking EMRs with laboratory values and medication administration records in outpatient settings similar in sophistication and design as are available in institutional settings.[5,6] Using the knowledge gained from decades of hospital experience with health IT, steps to reduce medication errors should be implemented in ambulatory settings just as they are in institutional settings. Since most ambulatory patients receive care on an outpatient basis, the need is just as crucial for these patients as is for institutional setting patients.[6,7]

What Are the Necessary Components for Optimal Use and e-Prescribing Success?

Existing software, hardware systems, handheld computer device technology, and a series of necessary steps all intersect to provide support for e-prescribing platforms and systems and subsequent needs.

Use of Personal Digital Assistants (PDAs)

The convenience and ease of use of PDAs is a positive feature that can encourage physician usage of e-prescribing.[8] Physicians can theoretically analyze pricing, drug interactions, dosing, contraindications, and off-label indications through e-prescribing accoutrements. Whether or not all of these features will have appeal to a busy physician is an empirical question to be tested.

Pyramid for Technology Implementation

Scalise describes an e-prescribing pyramid with 6 levels necessary for building an adequate e-prescribing platform for optimal use and application from the ground up.[8] The levels in descending order of sophistication are as follows:[8(p.46)]

- Level 1: Integration with a more complete electronic health record
- Level 2: Stand-alone prescription writer, with no medication history or supporting data
- Level 3: A database of basic information, such as allergies, demographics, and formulary information, which can then be used to generate alerts
- Level 4: Medication management: long-term tracking and monitoring of each patient's active medications
- Level 5: Connectivity among practices, pharmacies, payers, pharmacy benefit managers, intermediaries and patients
- Level 6: Electronic drug reference only (no prescribing capability)

Steps to Enable e-Prescribing

Halamka et al suggest 5 steps to enabling e-prescribing: (1) one-on-one training and support upon initial deployment, (2) strong marketplace sponsorship, (3) vendor marketing and outreach, (4) analyzing the workload impact upon physicians, and (5) estimating the need for a communitywide approach to implementation.[9]

Teich and Marchibroda have compiled a thorough report detailing necessary actions for a quick implementation of e-prescribing.[10] Please see **Table 5-1** for a listing of 12 items pertinent to e-prescribing, benefits, and needs for adoption on a widespread basis. This report, *Electronic Prescribing: Toward Maximum Value and Rapid Adoption*, published in 2004, remains the most comprehensive listing of the state of adoption regarding e-prescribing in the United States.[10] This report provides a useful blueprint to guide the implemention of e-prescribing systems.

TABLE 5-1 **Highlights of the *Electronic Prescribing: Toward Maximum Value and Rapid Adoption* Report**
1. According to varying research reports spanning many decades, errors and adverse drug events in ambulatory care errors can be common, serious, and many can be preventable.
2. Electronic prescribing holds the potential to improve safety, quality, efficiency, and cost. Studies that model outcomes suggest that the national savings from universal adoption could be as high as $27 billion.
3. Electronic prescribing systems are available in a variety of graduated levels. Systems at the highest levels of sophistication afford much greater opportunities for benefit, although all of the middle and higher levels convey some significant benefits. At present, the projections detailing differing levels of sophistication need empirical testing for the assurance of intended effects.
4. Despite the benefits of electronic prescribing, adoption is still modest. Current surveys estimate that between 5% and 18% of physicians and other clinicians are using electronic prescribing. Potential barriers to clinician adoption include start-up cost, lack of specific reimbursement for start-up and continuation, and fear of reduced efficiency in the practice.
5. The adoption and use of electronic prescribing should be encouraged through the deployment of appropriate incentives. These incentives will be critical to widespread adoption. Federal and private monetary incentives to encourage adoption will produce increases in physician uptake. Similar incentives may not be available for pharmacies who adopt e-prescribing technologies.
6. Continuing progress toward better-designed, more usable systems is likely to help adoption. As with any electronically mediated technology, upgrades and enhancements are commonplace.
7. Clinical decision support interventions should follow certain design principles for maximum acceptability and impact. This caveat has been followed in the marketplace.

(continues)

TABLE 5-1 *(Continued)*

---

8. Electronic communication offers numerous advantages: it is faster, more work-efficient, more secure, more reliable, less error-prone, and less prone to abuse than paper or fax prescriptions. Current barriers include expense, broadband availability, and variant standards. In addition, in some cases security and piracy concerns have stalled adoption.

---

9. Software should inform but not mandate a clinician's and patient's choice of medications and pharmacies. Patient confidentiality must also be protected. System override capabilities are in place with systems, but formulary and plan design stipulations may supersede prescriber or pharmacist intentions.

---

10. A number of enhancements in standards and vocabularies are needed to improve quality, efficiency, and to facilitate interoperability between the various electronic systems involved in the electronic prescribing process. Unifying state prescription-form standards, establishing a consistent "doctor-level" drug vocabulary, and standardizing formulary information are among the highest needs. These suggestions are being institutionalized in current and planned for systems.

---

11. Careful management of the initial use period in any practice is essential. Access to registration, schedule, and prior medication information is important. The uploading of patient data may be the key limiting step for adoption for many physicians. The question is, who will pay for or do the work necessary for system implementation? Entering patients manually (if necessary) into systems will be cumbersome, expensive, and time consuming.

---

12. Integration of electronic prescribing with an overall electronic health record adds value in a number of ways. Many lessons about adoption of electronic prescribing can be applied to the widespread adoption of robust, connected electronic health records as well. Again, many of these suggested enhancements are empirical questions.

Adapted from: Teich JM, Marchibroda JM. *Electronic Prescribing: Toward Maximum Value and Rapid Adoption* (A Report of the Electronic Prescribing Initiative). Washington, DC: eHealth Initiative; April 14, 2004.

Enhancing the Accuracy of Drug Prescribing

Authors have detailed the drug use quality enhancements that can occur with e-prescribing implementation.[11,12] The accuracy and increase in quality of care provided are real, tangible outcomes of e-prescribing technology. Bell and Friedman have suggested several benefits for e-prescribing:[11]

- Transmission of orders accurately among prescribers, pharmacies, and health plans, thereby reducing prescribing errors

- Help for physicians in adhering to guidelines (this might be evidence-based medicine guidelines, or formulary guidelines)
- Provision of a better mechanism to monitor patients' responses to treatment
- Help for providers to stay current with information on treatment protocols and varying aspects of new medications

In recommendations following a national retrospective study with the Veterans Affairs (VA) Health System, e-prescribing has been suggested as an intervention that can help to curb medication errors in outpatient VA settings.[12] After adjusting for diagnoses, dose, and duration, inappropriate prescribing decreased from 33% to 23%. In the VA studies, pain relievers, benzodiazepines, antidepressants, and musculoskeletal agents constituted 61% of inappropriate prescribing.[12] Interventions targeted at prescriptions for pain relievers, benzodiazepines, antidepressants, and musculoskeletal agents may dramatically decrease inappropriate prescribing and improved patient outcomes; e-prescribing was noted to be one suggested helpful remedy for this misuse.[12]

Value-Added Aspects of e-Prescribing

There are many aspects of e-prescribing that provide great opportunities to further enhance the outcomes of drug therapy. Some of these options for enhancing drug use cannot be accomplished with current systems in place for prescribing and dispensing. Numerous monitoring aspects associated with e-prescribing that enable a more sophisticated opportunity to analyze include:

- Drug use contraindications
- Appropriate dosage requirements
- Evidence-based prescribing appropriateness
- Patient-specific drug use considerations
- Drug therapy options

Promotion of e-Prescribing

Promotional materials for e-prescribing software tout the ability that users will have to maintain complete medication and allergy history, to check for drug interactions and allergies, to check patient-specific formulary information, and to complete refill authorizations with just a few strokes of a keypad.[13] Some newer releases will also include nursing notes, vital signs monitoring, physician order entry, medication schedules, and dispensing tracking. All this is coupled with electronic signature capability.[13]

Using e-Prescribing to Monitor Patient Medication Compliance and Persistence

Linking e-prescribing, EMRs, and associated electronically digitized information can enable the tracking of medication adherence and predictors of suboptimal adherence for populations and subpopulations of patients.[14,15] This capability can offer health care providers with additional information to better serve patient needs. This also enables an ability to monitor patient compliance and persistence on a population basis. Thus, a physician and pharmacist can identify a group or subgroup of patients and follow prescription refill compliance behavior.

This ability coupled with other efforts to monitor and enhance medication compliance are features that may impact the estimated 50% rate of medication compliance present in the United States. Initial compliance refers to patients initially filling prescriptions after they have been written by prescribers. These prescriptions can conceivably be left at a pharmacy for filling by patients or patient representatives or phoned or faxed by physicians or physician representatives to a pharmacy. Initially noncompliant prescriptions are never filled and/or picked up for initial patient use. Initially noncomplied rates in the United States are estimated to be between 3% and 20%. e-Prescribing systems can identify immediately those prescriptions that are initially not complied with.

Cost Issues and Ramifications

e-Prescribing has been suggested to be cost-effective in reducing prescribing errors and increasing the accuracy of medication use prescribing and dispensing. Muñoz, while pointing out the benefits of e-prescribing, noted that a shift by physicians and pharmacies from handwritten to email drug prescriptions could save $29 billion.[16] e-Prescribing can be cost-effective for all size practices, but reports in the literature point to a more rapid return on investment in larger practices.[17]

As Is to Be Expected, Problems Remain

e-Prescribing will simply not be the be-all and end-all of factors leading to pre-scribing errors. Electronic prescribing is not the cure-all for all medication errors or inappropriate drug prescribing. In a study of pediatric patients and the occur-rence of medication errors, potential error rates were not lower with the institu-tion of e-prescribing.[18]

Costs and Lack of Cost Effectiveness

Articles have summarized some of the CMS efforts to incorporate e-prescribing in the United States. Not all of those providing input have been overwhelmingly positive.[19] The Medical Group Management Association (MGMA) was one of several industry groups that weighed in, filing a generally supportive 14-page memorandum that included several "yes, but" caveats.[19]

The MGMA has contended that the benefits of e-prescribing are not cost-effective. MGMA also has called for federal tax credits, tax-sheltered technology savings accounts, and forgivable federal loans for medically underserved areas to provide incentives for physicians investing in health care IT.[19]

The American Medical Association has noted in publications that "some physicians don't want to 'bite off more than they can chew,' so e-prescribing (eRx) is an attractive first step into Health Information Technology (HIT)."[20(p.1)] The start-up costs for e-prescribing systems, and expansions of such, may also be a deterrent for some physicians.

Better Control of Risky or At-Risk Drugs

Controlled Substances

One tangible benefit suggested to occur with implementation of e-prescribing is a safety issue regarding prescribing and dispensing controlled substances. Berliner indicates that e-prescribing will help address the abuse of controlled sub-stances by some patients.[21]

Teratogenic Drugs

Teratogenic drugs would also be better controlled in at-risk females if these drugs had accompanying warning notes that could be alerts in e-prescribing systems and be evident when these drugs were inappropriately prescribed for pregnant patients.[22]

More Accurate Dosing with Chemotherapy

Roscoe et al note that contemporary cancer treatment requires a multidisciplinary approach in order to ensure the safe prescribing and administration of chemotherapy.[23] Using e-prescribing with drugs having a narrow therapeutic index can provide monitoring, other safety features, and appropriate dosing and spacing of chemotherapeutic agents with more ease than offered via traditional prescribing systems.

More Control of Black Box Warning Affected Drugs

Another benefit of e-prescribing would be alerting systems for avoidance of prescribing drugs with a black box warning to patients for whom the use would be contraindicated.[24] These types of drugs would have cautionary warnings evident when prescribed for inappropriate patients via e-prescribing.

Summation of Benefits

This chapter has presented numerous benefits that would accrue to the use of e-prescribing on a large scale. Proponents for e-prescribing have been vocal in promoting the technology. These supporters have relied upon political, quality of care, economic, and therapeutic rationales for supporting e-prescribing.

e-Prescribing Considerations

e-Prescribing occurs when the physician enters prescription information electronically, which is then automatically transmitted to the pharmacy for dispensing. There is nothing that the patient needs to do other than simply go to the pharmacy to pick up the medication. This has the potential to decrease errors in prescribing and dispensing and make it easier for the patient to comply. The Medicare Prescription Drug, Improvement, and Modernization Act of 2003 includes e-prescribing as a component to be standardized by 2009.

Final Caution

Currently, we live in an age when IT is eclipsing our ability to properly monitor what is being transmitted and to whom. Compliance interventions can be developed with the technology available; however, important safeguards need to be in place to ensure that only those who need to access such information are the ones with such access. Computerization of medical and pharmacy records affords providers and institutions unique ways to store voluminous amounts of health data without the expansive storage that was necessary in the past. Unless safeguards are enacted, the transfer of information can have a negative impact in addition to the intended positive effects.

Concluding Considerations

According to a Pharmaceutical Care Management Association (PCMA) report conducted by the Gorman Health Group, the following items are pertinent to e-prescribing considerations:[25]

- Government options to increase e-prescribing could reduce federal health expenditures by up to $29 billion over the next decade and help physicians to prevent nearly 1.9 million adverse drug events (ADEs) over the same time period, where individuals otherwise would have been sickened, hospitalized, or killed by serious medication errors.

- Approximately 70 percent of the safety and savings advantages of e-prescribing result from doctors being given immediate access to patient medication histories, safety alerts, preferred drug options, and pharmacy options so that they can better counsel patients on safe and affordable choices *before* prescriptions are transmitted to the pharmacy.

- Government action—including the three options below—could potentially expand e-prescribing to encompass nearly 80 percent of prescriptions by 2017—more than *double* the share of prescriptions expected to flow through e-prescribing systems by that time if no government action is taken.
  - Option 1—Requirement and Incentive: Implementing *a requirement* that e-prescribing is used for all Part D prescriptions by 2010 *combined with annual incentives* for participating physicians equal to 1 percent of their allowed Medicare payments could reduce 2008–2017 federal healthcare costs by $26 billion and help physicians avoid 1.9 million adverse drug events over the next ten years.

○ Option 2—Requirement Only: Implementing *only a requirement* that all Part D prescriptions be written electronically by 2010 could reduce 2008–2017 federal healthcare costs by $29 billion and help physicians avoid 1.6 million adverse drug events over the next ten years.

○ Option 3—Incentives Only: Implementing *only incentives* for participating physicians equal to 1 percent of their allowed Medicare payments could reduce 2008–2017 federal healthcare costs by $2 billion and help physicians avoid 300,000 adverse drug events over the next ten years.

Finally, as noted in this chapter, tangible benefits of e-prescribing include immediate access to:

- Prescription eligibility
- Formulary and benefits
- Medication history information for patients

In addition, patients can optimize their prescription drug benefits and choose any pharmacy of their choice. Health benefit plans can improve formulary compliance, achieve more efficient generic/therapeutic interchange, and reduce administrative time and cost.

References

1. Institute of Medicine. *Preventing Medication Errors*. Washington, DC: The National Academies; 2006.
2. Gingrich N, Kerry J. e-Prescriptions. *Wall Street Journal–Eastern Edition*. November 16, 2007:A20.
3. Department of Health and Human Services. *Health Information Technology: American Health Information Community*. Available at: http://www.hhs.gov/healthit/community/background. Accessed May 26, 2008.
4. McGee MK. Boost for e-prescriptions. *InformationWeek*. August 16, 2004:14.
5. Davis RL. Computerized physician order entry systems: the coming of age for outpatient medicine. *PLOS Medicine*. 2005;2(9):290.
6. Davis RL. Potential medication dosing errors in outpatient pediatrics. *J Pediatr*. 2005; 147(6):761–767.
7. Adubofour K, Keenan C, Daftary A, Nesah-Adubofour J, Dachman WD. Strategies to reduce medication errors in ambulatory practice. *J Nat Med Assoc*. 2004;96(12): 1558–1564.

8. Scalise D. The case for e-prescribing. *Hosp Health Net.* 2007;81(2):45–50.

9. Halamka J, Aranow M, Ascenzo C, et al. e-Prescribing collaboration in Massachusetts: early experiences from regional prescribing projects. *J Am Med Inform Assoc.* 2006;13: 239–244.

10. Teich J, Marchibroda J. *Electronic Prescribing: Toward Maximum Value and Rapid Adoption* (A Report of the Electronic Prescribing Initiative). Washington, DC: eHealth Initiative; 2004.

11. Bell DS, Friedman MA. e-Prescribing and the Medicare Modernization Act of 2003. *Health Aff.* 2006;24(5):1159–1169.

12. Pugh MJ, Fincke BG, Bierman A, et al. Potentially inappropriate prescribing in elderly veterans: are we using the wrong drug, wrong dose, or wrong duration? *J Am Geriatr Soc.* 2005;53(8):1282–1289.

13. Behavioral Health Monitor. Electronic prescribing capability. *Behav Health Manag.* 2006;26(1):38.

14. Grant RW, Devita N, Singer D, Meigs J. Polypharmacy and medication adherence in patients with type 2 diabetes. *Diabetes Care.* 2003;26(5):1408–1412.

15. Geers H, Blaey C, Egberts A, Bouvy M, Heerdink E. Early identification of long-term poor adherence in ambulatory patients. *Ann Pharmacother.* 2006;40(12):2277–2278.

16. Muñoz SS. Rx by e-mail may save $29 billion. *Wall Street Journal–Eastern Edition.* April 15, 2004:D7.

17. Corley ST. Electronic prescribing: a review of costs and benefits. *Top Health Info Manag.* 2003;24(1):29–38.

18. McPhillips HA, Stille CJ, Smith D, Hecht J, et al. Potential medication dosing errors in outpatient pediatrics. *J Pediatr.* 2006;147(6):761–767.

19. Conn J. Rx for e-prescribing. *Mod Healthc.* 2005;35(16):33.

20. American Medical Association. *e-Prescribing Functionality.* Available at: http://www .ama-assn.org/ama/pub/category/16704.html. Accessed May 29, 2008.

21. Berliner N. The case for e-prescribing: the electronic medical record: part 2. *Pharm Rep.* 2006;36(10):32.

22. Schwarz EB, Maselli J, Norton M, Gonzales R. Prescription of teratogenic medications in United States ambulatory practices. *Am J Med.* 2005;118:1240–1249.

23. Roscoe JC, Goransson E, Slancar M, Smith J, Taylor S, Tyson S. A multidisciplinary approach to ensure safety in the prescribing and administration of chemotherapy. *J Onc Pharm Pract.* 2000;6(2):60–63.

24. Lasser KE, Seger DL, Yu DT, et al. Adherence to black box warnings for prescription medications in outpatients. *Arch Int Med.* 2006;166(3):338–344.

25. Gorman Health Group. *Options to Increase e-Prescribing in Medicare: Reducing Medication Errors and Generating up to $29 Billion in Savings for the Federal Government.* Washington, DC: Author; 2007.

SIX

What e-Prescribing Can Help Solve and What It Cannot Accomplish

Introduction

e-Prescribing systems were first used in the mid to late 1970s. Their prominence became more significant when, in 1999, the U.S. Institute of Medicine endorsed their use as a way to diminish the 98,000 hospitalized patients who die yearly from medication errors. Often when we are presented with a new technology or an improved upgrade to existing options, there is a sense that problems will be made much easier to solve. With the case of drug use problems, there are many variables that impact medication errors, adverse effects, and problems with patient compliance. e-Prescribing can help to ameliorate some of these vexing problems, but it will not solve them all. Let's explore what might be amenable to change and what may not be impacted by the new technology of e-prescribing.

What e-Prescribing Cannot Do

Much of the many positive components of e-prescribing will be described here shortly. However, it is important to first discuss some things that e-prescribing should not be expected to do, or even to be considered as a solution for several systemic problems, in the U.S. drug use process.

Consideration of Improper Access and Resultant Impacts

Abuses have been noted when patients are unaware of accessed information, often for marketing purposes. Examples might be patient contacts identified through data mining, with the data subsequently sold—all this done without the patient's knowledge or, most importantly, consent to do so. Along with the many positive features and outcomes associated with e-prescribing, there are cautions to be observed. With the powerful collection of personal health data, abuses can occur if attendant safeguards are not in place. Wingfield et al note that the access of electronic patient medication records allows for data mining, sometimes for economic and not therapeutic endpoints.[1] In both the United Kingdom National Health Service (NHS) and the U.S. PBM industry, collection of data will allow for population level assessment of drug outcomes, both good and bad. However, a clarification of the rights of an organization versus individual control over access to archived information will need to be accomplished.[2,3] For example, there have been instances when a new drug has been promoted to patients who were unaware of how they were identified or singled out.[4]

Errors Occurring with e-Prescribing

Paradoxically, drug errors can occur with e-prescribing, which is widely touted to decrease drug errors. In an analysis of a serious drug error with intravenous potassium chloride ordered via CPOE, authors characterized errors in several converging aspects of the drug ordering process: confusing on-screen laboratory results review, system usability difficulties, user training problems, and suboptimal clinical system safeguards that all contributed to a serious dosing error.[5] As with any technology—new or old—all problems will not be solved by implementing e-prescribing either. In a 2005 *Washington Post* column, Boodman noted:[6(p.HE01)]

> Computerized drug ordering systems have been regarded as essential in reducing medication errors, the most prevalent and preventable kind of mistake that experts say affects an estimated 770,000 hospitalized patients annually. A review of death certificates from 1993 found that

drug errors killed nearly 7,400 patients, according to the Institute of Medicine (IOM).

Even with the positive features of e-prescribing, errors can still occur. Boodman points out, "Among the potential or actual mistakes researchers found occurred weekly: incorrect doses prescribed for patients; patients who failed to get medication in a timely manner because of computer-related problems; and difficulty determining which patient was supposed to get a drug that had been prescribed."[6(p.HE01)]

Impact on Formulary Adherence and Generic Drug Utilization

In one retrospective study, the influence of e-prescribing on formulary compliance and generic drug utilization was analyzed.[7] Ross et al found that for paid pharmacy claims from a large, national managed care organization, there were no differences found between predominantly e-prescribers and traditional prescribers in measures of formulary compliance or generic drug utilization.[7] The key word in the previous sentence is predominantly; the reader does not know if predominant means 50% or 100% e-prescribing activity by the physicians who e-prescribed in the study. As a more widespread adoption of e-prescribing by physicians occurs, rates of both formulary compliance and generic drug utilization undoubtedly will be expected to increase.

Varying Uptake by Community Pharmacy

It has been observed that from the current environment of e-prescribing small independent pharmacies are slow to upgrade their pharmacy management systems to accept e-prescriptions because of large fees charged by software vendors. Large chain pharmacies embrace e-prescribing at the corporate level, but local store support is low, and there is inadequate training of pharmacy staff.[8]

Varying Factors Influencing e-Prescribing

There have been impediments to the incorporation of e-prescribing into practices, facilities, or third-party programs. For example, physician resistance to change regarding e-prescribing, system cost, and inadequate planning to incorporate e-prescribing into the existing care process have been blamed for failures in introducing e-prescribing in health systems.[9]

What e-Prescribing Can Do

e-Prescribing has at various points been suggested to reduce clinical risk management, to provide operational efficiency, and to provide access to electronic patient records. Enabling clinical risk management can include reducing the occurrence of adverse drug events (ADEs). ADEs can be due to prescribing errors, wrong interpretation of orders, and dispensing errors. e-Prescribing can provide accurate prescriptions and records.

Reducing Adverse Drug Events

e-Prescribing provides decision support for the selection of prescription products; information about formularies, dosing, and frequency; checks for allergies to particular medications and for possible drug interactions; avoidance of therapeutic duplication; and maximum or minimum dose amounts.

Numerous Benefits of e-Prescribing

Various authors have noted that e-prescribing systems can provide computer-based support for creation, transmission, dispensation, and the monitoring of drug therapies. In various countries, these systems have been shown in certain circumstances to increase both the safety and quality of patient care.[10–15] CDSS and CPOE have made impacts on medications errors and have been promoted as techniques to make huge inroads on medication errors.[16] In the May 2005 issue of *JMCP*, McMullin et al found that e-prescribing that included a CDSS was associated with significant drug cost savings and reduction in the proportion of high-cost drugs in 8 therapeutic categories that were the target of CDSS messages to prescribers.[17] Thus, an e-prescribing system with a CDSS can influence prescribing and produce drug cost savings.[17]

Runaway Costs in the U.S. Health Care System

Spending on drugs as a percentage of what was spent on health care in total increased slightly from 2006 to 2007 from 10.07% to 10.14%.[18] Drivers for the significant costs of medications include increased technologies available, increasing numbers of patient and prescriptions per patient, and number of seniors taking advantage of the Medicare Part D Drug Benefit. Generic drug use accounts for over 63% of prescriptions filled in the United States, but as a percentage of expenditures on drugs in total remains 20%.[19] Brand-name drug purchases fuel the increase in spending on drugs as evidenced by these data.[19]

One of the tangible benefits of e-prescribing in third-party programs is the potential to reduce excess spending on drugs that are not on plan formularies, to reduce spending on drugs for which generic substitutes are available, and to reduce the number of drugs prescribed inappropriately. Third-party plans include prescription drug plans, Medicare Advantage plans, and Medicaid plans that have formulary and generic option warnings that indicate to the prescriber and/or dispenser that a certain drug prescribed may not be appropriate.

Several segments of e-prescribing systems will enable drugs to be used more appropriately and thus less expensively. Physicians will have alerts about formulary acceptability or lack thereof when entering specific drugs for patients, and pharmacists will have computer prompts that will serve as a gatekeeper for nonformulary, expensive, and inappropriately prescribed drugs (drug interaction, drug disease, drug dosage, or drug dosage form warnings). These prompts, when responded to appropriately, will help stem some of the drug expenses in the system that have been rising so precipitously from year to year.

e-Prescribing as a Means to Enhance Quality

Bell and colleagues note that e-prescribing may substantially improve health care quality.[20] Despite the complexity involved in evaluating systems, Bell et al suggest developing a conceptual framework when evaluating needs and possible e-prescribing solutions.[20] They point to a series of 14 options that e-prescribing can help address:[20(p.64)]

1. Patient selection or identification
2. Diagnosis selection and diagnosis-based reminders
3. Medication selection menus
4. Safety alerts
   a. Drug-choice errors, including allergies
   b. Allergies drug: drug interactions
   c. Drug: disease interactions
   d. Drug: lab (renal, hepatic function)
   e. Body size, age

5. Formulary alerts and formulary adherence
6. Dosage calculation
   a. Dosage errors
7. Data transmission to inpatient, retail, and/or mail-order pharmacy
8. Physician in-office dispensing
   a. Drug-choice errors
9. Patient education materials, coordination of education activities
10. Medication administration aids
11. Refill and renewal reminders
    a. Outpatient adherence
12. Corollary orders (e.g., for monitoring tests)
13. Automated patient questionnaires to detect adverse effects; other structured follow-up communication
14. Alerts for patients' failure to refill (This refers to the ability to see if patients do or do not refill prescriptions in a timely fashion.)
    a. Patient adherence

Ability to Detect Fraudulent Patient Activity

Another measure to improve quality is the ability to identify providers from whom patients seek care. This measure to enhance quality, and one that would be controlled through e-prescribing, is a fraud detection capability that would be built into every e-prescribing system. Patients could not "shop around" for numerous physicians to write prescriptions for them. This has been a problem for decades in the United States, as some patients have attempted to see numerous physicians with the intent of obtaining many prescriptions from differing doctors. These abuses by patients have resulted in multiple prescribing of drugs of abuse, antibiotics, antidepressants, and other drugs; e-prescribing will help to eliminate this problem. Interestingly enough, prior to e-prescribing and the benefits accrue to its use, other attempts to diminish and/or stop this serious problem have all fallen short. At various times, people had tried to use duplicate or triplicate prescription pads (paper) to try to stem the abuse—none of which worked to the same extent that e-prescribing will. At present in 2008, tamper-proof prescriptions are being required in Medicaid programs, as is the case in some states regardless of payer.

Systems in Place to Enable e-Prescribing for Optimal Effects

The electronic architecture and backbone necessary to enable e-prescribing are in place at present in the United States. Major systems that have been effective in transmitting information from physicians' software to pharmacies and from pharmacies to PBMs and insurers have been shown to provide all the benefits available from e-prescribing. Hale has noted:[21(p.1)]

> The electronic prescribing process also requires intermediaries for Data Transfer to communicate the prescription information between the software system in the physician offices to the system in the pharmacies, and also for transmitting information to and from PBMs and health plans. Currently, SureScripts® is the major provider of communication between physician office software and pharmacies and RxHub® is the major provider of secure communication between the pharmacies and physician software with PBMs and health plans.

Viewing e-Prescribing with a Systems Approach

A systems approach or fail-safe analysis has been advocated to view prescribing safety and to avoid prescribing misadventures in similar fashion to other high risk activities in society.[22] Don Berwick, a noted scholar on medication errors, and coauthors have suggested that protecting patient safety can be adapted from other high risk industries, such as civil aviation, nuclear power, and other industries.[22] Berwick and colleagues provide a framework to guide quality improvement that includes 5 systemic barriers to safe patient care and 3 problems that are specific to health care. The systemic barriers arise from the discretion permitted for workers, worker autonomy, a craftsmanship mindset (that needs to transition to a mindset of equivalent actors), insufficient system-level (senior leadership) arbitration to optimize safety strategies, and the need for simplification.[22]

Foreign Experience with e-Prescribing

Sweden

Because of a one-payer system of health insurance and other factors regarding health professionals, EMRs are widely available in Sweden. In addition, data and information is accessible. The Swedes have found:[23(p.2)]

- An increase in data security and quality of prescription writing and processing since there is a continuous chain of information between the physician and/or hospital and the pharmacy.

- A 15% reduction in prescribing errors has been realized since both the physician and pharmacist are working with the same information.

- The efficiencies derived from time savings attributable to e-prescribing have been applied to other patient care needs.

- Health providers, hospitals, physicians, and pharmacists benefit from:
  - Avoidance of illegible prescriptions, i.e., the pharmacist does not have to call the physician to verify what is on the prescription
  - Time saved by doctors and nurses using e-prescribing is considerable
  - Reduced risk of fraud and prescription falsification, which previously was problematic
  - Avoidance of duplicate prescriptions, which were necessary to replace lost or misplaced prescriptions

The United Kingdom

Researchers in the United Kingdom have conducted a thorough analysis of e-prescribing in several health care settings.[24] When evaluating e-prescribing in multiple settings, Barber et al listed the following as key lessons learned from their research:[24(p.11)]

- Electronic prescribing (EP) needs to be addressed as a "sociotechnical" innovation, not just a technical solution "there for the taking."

- An extended implementation period needs to be resourced to provide support and to help good new practices embed.

- Emergent change should be expected and be managed. This can be quite profound, for example, EP could lead to a reduction in interaction with patients and between other professionals.

- Technical systems are never perfect; they should continue to be developed both to improve performance and to embody new and changing understanding.

- Software should be specified so it is possible to adapt it locally, and so that the data held are easily accessible for multiple purposes.

- Decision support is not straight forward; the purpose and limitations of decision support needs to be clear to all concerned.

Barber et al conclude:[24(p.136)]

> Our findings, taken overall, tentatively suggest that for every 100 prescriptions written in a hospital there will be around 10 errors; the introduction of an electronic prescribing system, at the current stage of development, would avoid two or three of them.

Canada

The equivalent of the FDA in the United States in Canada is Health Canada. In Canada, Health Canada has been involved in e-prescribing. The Canada Health Infoway is a Canadian government effort to enable EMRs to be available in Canada; it has worked to develop standards to enable e-prescribing activities between prescribers and pharmacists. The standards are required to support amendments under the regulation-making authority of the *Food and Drug Act*, the *Controlled Drug and Substance Act*, and possibly the *Personal Information Protection and Electronic Documents Act (PIPEDA)*. Health Canada has interacted with interested parties along the way. These key stakeholders, such as pharmacy and health practitioner regulatory bodies and federal/provincial/territorial government institutions, have worked together on such efforts.

Similar U.S. Food and Drug Administration Efforts

The U.S. FDA has initiatives underway to encourage e-prescribing. In a speech before the Urban Institute on November 12, 2003, the then-FDA commissioner Dr. Mark McClellan noted:[25]

> For example, to ensure that up-to-date drug information will be available to clinicians at the point of care, FDA is developing its new structured medical product labels in conjunction with new standards to make this label fully electronic, through our DailyMed program. The goal is to give the kind of IT-based support systems for good prescribing access to FDA's full, up to date database on the evidence on approved medical product use.
>
> FDA has worked with the National Library of Medicine to maintain a comprehensive inventory of these "electronic drug labels" and will

distribute this information free of charge to providers and IT vendors, possibly along with other useful information from medical studies. This will serve as the definitive source of drug information, since it will represent the body of evidence reviewed and approved by FDA.

The National Institutes of Health (NIH) Web site DailyMed provides information about marketed drugs in the United States. The Web site states:[26]

DailyMed provides high quality information about marketed drugs. This information includes FDA approved labels (package inserts). This Web site provides health information providers and the public with a standard, comprehensive, up-to-date, look-up and download resource of medication content and labeling as found in medication package inserts.

Other information about prescription drugs may also be available. NLM regularly processes data files uploaded from FDA's system and provides and maintains this Web site for the public to use in accessing the information. Additional information about medicines is available on NLM's MedlinePlus Web site, http://www.nlm.nih.gov/medlineplus/medicines.html.

Finland

e-Prescribing has been implemented in Finland for several years. The problems identified in the United States as concerns also were prominent in the inauguration of the Finnish system.[27] There are numerous factors that have enabled e-prescribing to be implemented in foreign systems, such as the Finnish system:

- A one-payer health care insurance system
- EMRs
- Enhanced communication between physicians and pharmacists
- Seamless interactions between prescribers, dispensers, and health care institutions

U.S. Progress

A relative lack of any of these points will not preclude a gradual implementation of e-prescribing in the United States. In fact, these foreign systems can help those seeking e-prescribing implementation in the United States to avoid pitfalls and problem areas. The United States can learn much from these foreign examples of forays into e-prescribing.

Impact of Existing Technology on e-Prescribing

The emergence of the enhanced sophistication of handheld and wireless transmission of data will also stimulate the additional application of e-prescribing. This technology factor is important as are the time, error, and economic savings that e-prescribing can provide.[28] Curtiss notes:[28(p.420)]

> In the last year, Blackberry and other wireless communication devices have been breaking down barriers of resistance to change. The ubiquitous and low effort features of this technology will transfer to clinician prescribing, and rather than resisting e-prescribing, clinicians will be demanding it. Yet, it will remain necessary to spend money on new and upgraded system software to integrate e-prescribing with the electronic medical record to overcome electronic silos of data that reside in pharmacies, at pharmacy benefit managers, or in data warehouses and are not available to clinicians at the point of care. What will shorten the timeline between the reality of today and the inevitability of tomorrow is studious examination of the work of pioneers in adapting and implementing IT solutions in health care settings.

Gaps That Inhibit e-Prescribing Uptake

Current physician use of e-prescribing is estimated to be between 3% and 18%, depending on definitions. Ridinger notes that an e-prescribing system would ensure optimization of safety, quality, and cost-benefit of therapeutics in clinical practice but is only one critical component of broader initiatives being implemented to optimize health care delivery.[27]

Gaps Also Occur in Many Places in Health Care
Curtiss has suggested:[28(p.419)]

> The gap between expectations and reality is large nearly everywhere one looks in health care. While there are success stories, more often, the truth

is that success stories are limited to distinct subsets or compartments of the health care system; use of the IT solution is voluntary by clinicians, thereby undermining the value of digital information because it is not complete; the IT system is plagued with errors,[29] or a backlash occurs among clinicians who find the new IT system burdensome rather than helpful.[30] The solution to IT over promises is lower expectations for IT proposals to meet the need for safety, quality, and administrative efficiency in health care.

[Author's Note: The two secondary references in the above extract are Ridinger[29] and Curtiss.[30]]

More Limitations of e-Prescribing

There are a number of problems within the prescribing, dispensing, and drug use processing that will not be influenced by e-prescribing. Some of these factors are drug specific, patient specific, or system specific in nature. Patient medication noncompliance and persistence, over-the-counter (OTC) drug misuse, occurrence of adverse drug reactions, prescribing errors, and/or dispensing errors are commonplace. No systems yet devised or planned can totally eliminate these problems from negatively influencing appropriate drug use in the U.S. health care system.[31] Let's explore what some of the problems related to drug use are that cannot be remedied by e-prescribing.

Fundamental Flaws in Drug Use Process

There are fundamental flaws in the drug use process in the United States. Medication compliance hovers around 50%, and prescription drug misuse is rampant. OTC medications are misused. Adverse drug events occur (many of which are preventable). Antibiotic misuse has led to drug resistant strains of many bacteria. Despite recent changes to Medicare, many patients remain uninsured with respect to prescription medications. e-Prescribing will not by itself impact these and other systemic medication-related error producing system segments.

Increase in Self-Medication
Self-medication can be broadly defined as a decision made by a patient to consume a drug without the explicit approval or direction of a health professional.

Self-medication in and of itself has many positive aspects with many benefits to patients when done appropriately. The self-medication activities of patients increased dramatically in the late 20th century and on into the 21st century. Many contemporary developments have continued to fuel this increase:

- There are ever increasing locations from which to purchase OTC medications.
- There have been many medications switched to OTC classification from prescription-only classification in the last 50 years.
- Patients are increasingly becoming comfortable with self-diagnosis and self-selection of OTC remedies.

These important OTC therapeutic agents, that just happen to be sold and used without a prescription, will not be captured in e-prescribing systems. They are purchased by consumers, in some instances, without their health professionals being aware of the use. Important impacts on disease states and deleterious effects on other drugs, which are prescribed, can cause problems. For example, using aspirin, which has blood thinning properties, with a drug that is prescribed, such as sodium warfarin, can lead to dangerous bleeding episodes if used together. Using nonprescription analgesics, such as acetaminophen, with prescription analgesics also containing acetaminophen can be problematic. These duplications will not be addressed or influenced by e-prescribing.

Direct-to-Consumer Advertising

Direct marketing of drugs by pharmaceutical manufacturers to consumers has also contributed to rising prescription costs. Direct-to-consumer (DTC) advertising for prescription drugs doubled in the recent past, from $1.1 billion in 1997 to $2.7 billion in 2001.[32] Estimates for spending on DTC advertising in 2005 is $4.2 billion.[33] As drugs have been switched from prescription to OTC status, the advertising and promotion of these newly classified OTC drugs has increased as well.

Systems Cannot Indicate Where Consumers Obtain Medications

Although pharmacists are seen as the gatekeepers for patients to obtain prescription drugs, patients can also obtain prescription medications from other pharmacies and/or from dispensing physicians. Patients may also borrow from friends, relatives, or even casual acquaintances. In addition, patients obtain OTC medications from physicians through prescriptions, on advice from pharmacists, through self-selection, or through the recommendations of friends or acquaintances. Through all of this, it must be recognized that both formal (structural) and informal (pervasive) system components are at play. Pharmacists or physicians may or may not be consulted regarding the use of medications. In some cases, health professionals are unaware of the drugs patients are taking. In addition, herbal remedies or health supplements may be taken without the knowledge or input of a health professional.

As an example, consider the patient medication profiling capability of most pharmacists currently in place and those that will continue to be enabled by e-prescribing. Computerization of patient medication records is commonplace in pharmacies. This computerization allows for the following:

- Ease in billing third-party prescription programs
- Maintenance of drug allergy information
- Drug use review
- Notification of drug interactions
- Aid in meeting the Omnibus Budget Reconciliation Act of 1990 (OBRA '90) requirements for patient counseling, drug use review, and estimation of appropriateness of therapy

This computerization permits drug-related information to be easily entered, retained, and retrieved; however, OTC medications are rarely entered into such records (one exception may be OTC drugs prescribed by physicians and dispensed through a prescription by pharmacists). This exclusion of a whole class of drugs from the monitoring programs of pharmacies may have a profound effect upon the ability of pharmacists to monitor the drug therapies of their patients. If the patient purchases the OTC medication in the pharmacy, the pharmacist may have an idea of the drugs consumed; however, if OTC drugs are purchased in a nonpharmacy outlet, the pharmacist is completely unaware of many drugs a patient may be taking. Another factor adding to the complexity of the problem is that a patient also may utilize numerous pharmacies for varying prescription products. Thus, there is no one record repository for all medications a patient may be taking.

Lack of Insurance Coverage

External variables may greatly influence patients and their drug taking behaviors. Coverage for prescribed drugs allows those with coverage to obtain medications with varying cost-sharing requirements; however, many do not have insurance coverage for drugs or other health-related needs. It has been estimated that in 2006, 17% of Americans—approximately 47 million people—lacked health insurance for all or part of the year.[34] Certainly, these considerations have huge ramifications for how and when consumers obtain prescribed and OTC medications.

Those that do have health insurance have seen premiums rise drastically in the recent past, 8.4% to 11%.[34] Miller notes that in some cases employees are not just being asked to pay more for health insurance but to pay for it all.[35] Until this fundamental inequality is remedied through health policy changes and a differing perspective on insurance coverage for those currently uninsured is taken, no amount of sophisticated health IT implementations or e-prescribing enabling will impact this component of the health care delivery and access to care conundrum.

Adverse Drug Reactions

The occurrence of adverse drug reactions (ADRs) are sometimes frequent, sometimes sporadic, and more often than not, unpredictable. e-Prescribing can help to reduce ADRs if proper notation occurs in patients' records and is accessible electronically by prescribers and pharmacists. These notations indicating previous reactions, sensitivities, and alerts for drugs must be in place and not overridden by the prescribers and pharmacists.

The actual incidence of ADRs is unknown. Even in health care system institutions (hospitals and long-term care facilities) with elaborate health IT systems, ADRs still occur, despite sophisticated electronic systems that are available. There is not a foolproof system in place at present to report ADR occurrences. It is hoped that e-prescribing and associated systems will help to enable a more cohesive method of reporting and sharing ADR experiences.

Compliance

All involved in the drug use process need to understand patient compliance behaviors. Interventions cannot be tailored to meet patient therapeutic needs if patient drug taking behavior is unclear. Conversely, if patient drug-taking patterns are discernable, it is possible to help patients take medications as they should through varying types of compliance interventions. e-Prescribing systems are unlikely to impact individual patient behavior so as to enhance patient compliance and/or persistence.

Interventions that have been shown to be effective in enhancing compliance behavior include:

- Patient counseling (verbal or written)
- Specialized packaging (unit of use, unit dose, blister packs, specialized containers, and/or packaging of medications to be taken at the same time in the same unit of use containers)
- Varying refill reminders (letters mailed, e-mailed, telephone calls, etc.)
- Other types of specialized contacts

Obviously, if we cannot measure how patients are taking medications, it is not possible to formulate specialized aids to help patients take medications. Measurement of compliance can vary from mildly invasive (pill counts or questioning patients) to very invasive (blood level determination of compliance).

Pharmacists and providers can ask patients whether compliance is a problem with them, and the veracity of each of the responses is subject to verification. Blood levels can be measured, therapeutic outcomes can be measured, and indirect methods of estimating compliance (side effects, certain outcomes of drug use examined) can all be undertaken with varying assurances of accuracy.

Ultimately, the decision to comply or to not comply with recommendations, including prescription drug therapies, is a patient specific decision. e-Prescribing may streamline the process of providing the patient with the right drug, the correct dose, the appropriate dosing mechanism, and proper instructions for use. However, e-prescribing cannot enhance the decision to comply or not, or to help a caregiver enable compliance behavior for those for whom they provide care; at this point, the decision to comply or not is in the hands of the patient and/or caregiver.

Frank Errors

Despite elaborate and sophisticated health IT enabled e-prescribing, errors will continue to be made as long as humans are involved in health care. Physicians have the potential to make errors in prescribing (wrong patient; right patient—wrong drug, wrong dose, and/or wrong duration of therapy). Pharmacists are also capable of making errors in dispensing, labeling, misreading orders, or dispensing to the wrong patient. Patients also are able unfortunately to underdose, overdose, use the wrong drugs for the wrong length of time, or use the right drug for the wrong period of time.

Wrong Diagnoses

A startling 15% of diagnoses are estimated to be made in error.[35] Groopman further suggests that 80% of these errors are predictable based on how physicians go about diagnosing patients' maladies in such a compressed and hurried fashion.[36] e-Prescribing will not reverse this startling rate of inaccuracy. If the right drug is prescribed for the wrong diagnosis, the patient will always suffer.

Taking the Place of Face-to-Face Encounters?

There will always be a need for pharmacists to contact physicians via the telephone to deal with patient-related issues. They may include:

- Clarification of orders transmitted by physicians or physicians' representatives
- Follow-up on questionable orders from physicians
  - Determining if the patient is in fact the correct patient
  - Drug, dose, dosage form clarifications
- Dealing with therapeutic duplications, drug interactions (drug, food, supplement, etc.)
- Third-party insurance related concerns
- Clarification of refill instructions for repeating medication regimens
- Emergency contact when a physician is not in proximity to a computer, yet needs to phone in an order
- Suggestions for therapeutic alternatives when appropriate or required for one reason or another (insurance, patient needs, better choice of drug over what has been prescribed, etc.)

So, regardless of how well structured an e-prescribing system has been developed, there will always be situations where health care professionals will need to converse via phone contact as well as interact electronically.

Summary

e-Prescribing has unlimited potential to enhance the drug use process from prescribing to the point of patient delivery of medications. Error reduction, precise dosing, help in choosing the appropriate drug, and enhancement of quality are but a few of the potential and very real consequences of the uptake of e-prescribing. As is the case with any improvement in any industry, including the health care industry, the recognition of the many potential benefits and a thorough assessment of the issues that e-prescribing cannot address will bode well for all involved in the drug use process.

As noted in this chapter, e-prescribing will not solve all of the ills present in the U.S. prescribing, dispensing, and utilization processes for prescription drugs.

References

1. Wingfield J, Bissell P, Anderson C. The scope of pharmacy ethics—an evaluation of the international research literature, 1990–2002. *Soc Sci Med.* 2004,58:2383–2396.
2. O'Harrow R. Prescription sales, privacy fears: CVS giant share customer records with drug marketing firm. *Washington Post.* February 15, 1998:A1.
3. O'Harrow R. Giant food stops sharing customer data: prescription-marketing plan drew complaints. *Washington Post.* February 18, 1998:A1.
4. Ohliger PC. Are your medication records confidential? *Drug Benefit Trends.* 1999;11(2): 23–24.
5. Horsky J, Kuperman GJ, Patel VL. Comprehensive analysis of a medication dosing error related to CPOE. *J Am Med Inform Assoc.* 2005;12:377–382.
6. Boodman SG. Not quite fail-safe, computerizing isn't a panacea for dangerous drug errors. *Washington Post.* March 22, 2005:HE01.
7. Ross SM, Papshev D, Murphy EL, Sternberg DJ, Taylor J, Barg R. Effects of electronic prescribing on formulary compliance and generic drug utilization in the ambulatory care setting: a retrospective analysis of administrative claims data. *J Manag Care Pharm.* 2005;11(5):410–415.
8. Tcimpidis L, Rosenblatt M. Readers' perspectives. *Health Data Manag.* 2005;May:88.
9. Morrissey J. Harmonic divergence: Cedars-Sinai joins others in holding off on CPOE. *Mod Healthcare.* 2004;23:16.
10. Miller RA, Gardner RM, Johnson KB, Hripcsak G. Clinical decision support and electronic prescribing systems: a time for responsible thought and action. *J Am Med Inform Assoc.* 2005;12:403–409.
11. Bates DW, Leape LL, Cullen DJ. Effect of computerized physician order entry and a team intervention on prevention of serious medication errors. *JAMA.* 1998;280:1311–1316.
12. Bates DW, Teich JM, Lee J. The impact of computerized physician order entry on medication error prevention. *J Am Med Inform Assoc.* 1999;6:313–321.

13. Chertow GM, Lee J, Kuperman GJ. Guided medication dosing for inpatients with renal insufficiency. *JAMA*. 2001;286:2839–2844.

14. Potts AL, Barr FE, Gregory DF, Wright L, Patel NR. Computerized physician order entry and medication errors in a pediatric critical care unit. *Pediatrics*. 2004;113:59–63.

15. Chrischilles EA, Fulda TR, Byrns PJ, Winckler SC, Rupp MT, Chui MA. The role of pharmacy computer systems in preventing medication errors. *J Am Pharm Assoc (Wash)*. 2002;42:439–448.

16. Teich JM, Osheroff JA, Pifer EA, Sittig DF, Jenders RA, CDS Expert Review Panel. Clinical decision support. *J Am Med Inform Assoc*. 2007;14:141–145.

17. McMullin ST, Lonergan TP, Rynearson CS. 12-month drug cost savings related to use of an electronic prescribing system with integrated decision support in primary care. *J Manag Care Pharm*. 2005;11(4):322–332.

18. Poisal JA, Truffer C, Smith S, et al. Health spending projections through 2016: modest changes obscure part D's impact. *Health Aff*. 2007;26(2):w242–w253.

19. Kaiser Family Foundation. *Prescription Drug Trends, 2007* (Fact Sheet #3057-06). Washington, DC: Author; May 31, 2007. Available at: http://www.kff.org/rxdrugs/upload/3057_06.pdf. Accessed May 30, 2008.

20. Bell DS, Cretin S, Marken RS, Landman AB. A conceptual framework for evaluating outpatient electronic prescribing systems based on their functional capabilities. *J Am Med Inform Assoc*. 2004;11:60–70. Available at: doi:10.1197/jamia.M1374.

21. Hale P. *Electronic Prescribing Update: HIMSS Fact Sheet*. Available at: http://www.himss.org/content/files/CBO/Meeting7/ElectronicPrescribingUpdate.pdf. Accessed December 4, 2007.

22. Amalberti R, Auroy Y, Berwick D, Barach P. Five system barriers to achieving ultrasafe health care. *Ann Intern Med*. 2005;142(9):756–764.

23. European Commission Information Society and Media. *Apoteket and Stockholm County Council, Sweden—eRecept, an e-Prescribing Application*. Available at: http://ec.europa.eu/information_society/activities/health/docs/events/opendays2006/ehealth-impact-7-2.pdf. Accessed June 3, 2008.

24. Barber N, Franklin ED, Cornford T, Klecun E, Savage I. *Safer, Faster, Better? Evaluating Electronic Prescribing Report to the Patient Safety Research Programme* (Policy Research Programme of the Department of Health). London, United Kingdom: University of London; November 2006. Available at: http://eprints.pharmacy.ac.uk/763/1/Electronic PrescribingBarberFranklin.pdf. Accessed March 28, 2008.

25. McClellan MB. *Protecting and Advancing America's Health Through 21st Century Patient Safety* (Speech before the Urban Institute). November 12, 2003. Available at: http://www.fda.gov/oc/speeches/2003/urbaninstitute1112.html. Accessed March 7, 2008.

26. U.S. National Library of Medicine, National Institutes of Health. *DailyMed: Current Medication Information*. Available at: http://dailymed.nlm.nih.gov/dailymed/about.cfm. Accessed May 29, 2008.

27. Kansanaho H, Puumalainen I, Varunki M, Ahonen R, Airaksinen M. Implementation of a professional program in Finnish community pharmacies in 2000–2002. *Patient Educ Couns*. 2005;57(3):272–279.

28. Curtiss FR. Clinical, service, and cost outcomes of computerized prescription order entry. *J Manag Care Pharm*. 2005;11(4):353–355.

29. Ridinger MHT. The electronic prescription conundrum: why "e-Rx" isn't so "e-Z." *Clin Pharmacol Therap.* 2007;81:13–15. Available at: doi:10.1038/sj.clpt.6100022.

30. Curtiss FR. Why e-prescribe and the future of transforming data into information. *J Manag Care Pharm.* 2005;11(5):419–420.

31. Fernando B, Savelyich BS, Avery AJ, et al. Prescribing safety features of general practice computer systems: evaluation using simulated test cases. *BMJ.* 2004;328:1171–1172.

32. Jeffords JM. Direct-to-consumer drug advertising: you get what you pay for. *Health Aff.* 2004;Web exclusive:w253–w255. Available at: doi:10.1377/hlthaffw4.253.

33. Donohue JM, Cevasco M, Rosenthal MB. A decade of direct-to-consumer advertising of prescription drugs. *NEJM.* 2007;373(7):673–681.

34. Kaiser Family Foundation. *The Uninsured and Their Access to Health Care* (Fact sheet #1420-06). Washington, DC: Author; 2004.

35. Miller JL. *A Perfect Storm: The Confluence of Forces Affecting Health Care Coverage.* Washington, DC: National Coalition on Health Care; 2001.

36. Groopman J. *How Doctors Think.* New York: Houghton Mifflin; 2007.

SEVEN

Current Examples of e-Prescribing Options and Your Practice

Introduction

The focus of this chapter is on options for your consideration related to your practice and your needs relative to e-prescribing systems. Basically, e-prescribing relates to a physician's computer system being able to communicate with a computer system in pharmacies. These processes can be stand-alone or as a part of an existing electronic health record (EHR) system.

e-Prescribing Basics

Hale notes 2 components necessary for connectivity:[1(p.1)]

> The electronic prescribing process also requires intermediaries for Data Transfer to communicate the prescription information between the software system in the physician offices to the system in the pharmacies, and also for transmitting information to and from PBMs and health plans. Currently, SureScripts is the major provider of communication between

physician office software and pharmacies and RxHub is the major provider of communication between the pharmacies and physician software with PBMs and health plans.

Examples of RxHub Services

The following RxHub services, pictorial schematics, and descriptors are used with the permission of RxHub.[2] These products detailed below include RxHub PRN, RxHub SIG, RxHub MEDS, and RxHub Integration Services.

RxHub PRN

The RxHub PRN program:[3]

> . . . provides physicians in the ambulatory setting with patient-specific medication history and pharmacy benefit information at the point of care, giving the physician the ability to write an informed prescription. Through RxHub PRN, a prescriber can securely access prescription coverage information from participating payers and PBMs, using their practice's technology of choice, such as a computer, PDA or paper print-out that can be placed in the patient's chart. RxHub PRN is the only true end-to-end comprehensive ePrescribing solution today.
>
> With RxHub PRN physicians are able to:
>
> - Review patient concurrent medications and medication history information at the point of prescribing
> - Check patient group formulary coverage information at the point of prescribing
> - Communicate with RxHub Certified Payers through secure, industry standard transactions
>
> With RxHub PRN pharmacists are able to:
>
> - Check patient group eligibility and formulary coverage information at the point of dispensing

Please see **Figure 7-1** for a graphic descriptor of the RxHub PRN.

FIGURE 7-1   **RxHub PRN**

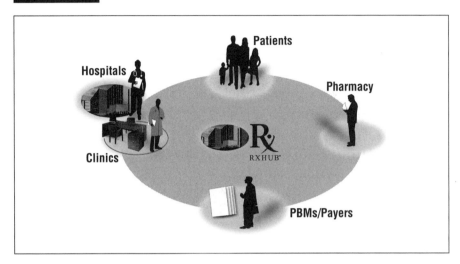

RxHub SIG

RxHub SIG provides direct, electronic delivery of a new prescription from a prescriber to the pharmacy of the patient's choice.[4] It also enables the pharmacy to send a renewal request or a change request to the prescriber and receive an immediate response.

RxHub SIG utilizes the NCPDP SCRIPT standard to:[4]

- Route new prescriptions from the prescriber to the patient's pharmacy of choice
- Route renewal requests from pharmacies to prescribers
- Route prescription change requests from pharmacies to prescribers

Please see **Figure 7-2** for a graphic descriptor of the RxHub SIG.

FIGURE 7-2 **RxHub SIG**

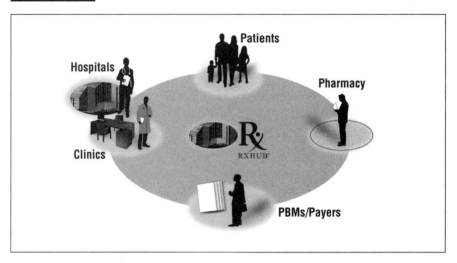

RxHub MEDS

RxHub MEDS contains the inpatient medication history function of RxHub.[5]

> RxHub MEDS provides physicians with convenient access to up-to-date medication history for patients they are treating in an inpatient setting. It starts with a directory service that routes the request to the appropriate data source. This directory, which currently contains the drug benefit eligibility status (but not the medication history) of more than 160 million covered lives (and continues to grow as we add new participants), is unprecedented in the health care industry. RxHub MEDS allows physicians who are treating patients in an inpatient setting to quickly access outpatient drug history, if the patient is an enrolled member of a health plan served by the PBMs. While drug history would be available only for members who choose to participate, many plans and employers have long sought to provide this type of information to physicians in inpatient settings to reduce medical errors. One of the major causes of medication errors in the hospital is the lack of complete patient information. As hospitals work to comply with JCAHO medication reconciliation requirements, RxHub MEDS provides that solution. RxHub is streamlining the acquisition and delivery of patient-specific information to help achieve safer outcomes.

With RxHub MEDS:

- Physicians can better avoid drug duplication and adverse drug events.
- Physicians have access to information that assists with prescribing, assessing a patient's current health condition, and recommending treatment.

Please see **Figure 7-3** for a graphic descriptor of the RxHub MEDS.

RxHub Integration Services

The final product we will discuss is the RxHub Integration Services.[6]

RxHub Integration Services provides a quick, secure, easy, cost-effective and certified connectivity for PBMs and Payers to the RxHub National Patient Health Information Network™, through the Cloverleaf Integration Suite operated by Quovadx, to provide a wide range of ePrescribing decision support information at the point of care.

Please see **Figure 7-4** for a graphic descriptor of the RxHub Integration Services.

FIGURE 7-3　**RxHub MEDS**

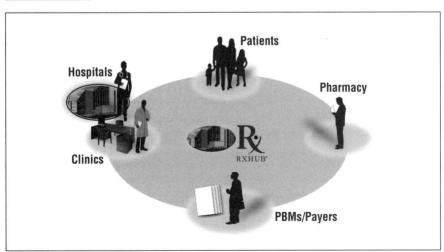

FIGURE 7-4 **RxHub Integration Services**

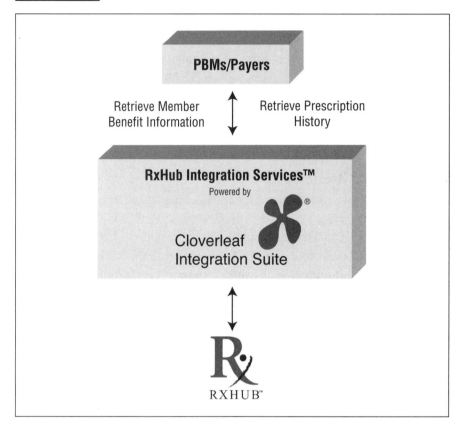

e-Prescribing Vendors

Please see **Table 7-1** for a listing of companies and products that are available for physicians to enable e-prescribing in their practices. This listing was updated as of June 2008; please note that frequent additions and deletions are commonplace with these technologies and applications.

What to Look for in e-Prescribing Vendor Options

SureScripts has developed a buyer's guide that is helpful to examine when considering what options for e-prescribing make the most sense for your practice.[7]

TABLE 7-1   e-Prescribing Companies and Products

Company	*Product*
ACS Heritage	CyberAccess v2.1.2
Allscripts	HealthMatics® EMR 4.8.1
Allscripts	TouchWorks v10.1.1
Allscripts/NEPSI	eRx NOW™ v1.0
ASP.MD	ASP.MD
athenahealth	athenaClinicals
Axolotl	Elysium v8.0.1
Blue Cross and Blue Shield of Alabama	InfoSolutions v2.0
BMA Enterprises	Chart Management System v1.2
Bond Medical	Bond EHR Clinician v2006
Cerner	Healthe Record v3.0
Cerner	PowerChart v M2007
ChartConnect	MedManager v6.8
Computer Programs and Systems, Inc. (CPSI)	Medical Practice v.14
DAW Systems	ScriptSure
digiChart OB-GYN	digiChart V 7.0
Doc-U-Chart	Doc-U-Scrip v4.0
DrFirst	DrFirst Rcopia v3.6.01
e-MDs	e-MDs Solution Series v6.1
eClinicalWorks, Inc.	eClinicalWorks v7.0
Eclipsys	Sunrise Ambulatory Care Manager 4.5 XA
eHealthSolutions	eHealthSolutions v4.4
EHS	CareRevolution V. 5.1
Epic	EpicWeb Spring 2007
Epic	EpicCare EMR Spring 2007
Glenwood Systems	Glace EMR v2
Gold Standard	eMPOWERx v3.09
H2H Solutions, Inc.	Digital Rx v1.5x
HealthPort	HealthPort Electronic Medical Records v9.0
Henry Schein Medical Systems	MicroMD EMR v 5.0
iMedica	Patient Relationship Manager V2007
iMedX	TurboRx
InstantDx	OnCallData v3.5
InteGreat	IC-Chart® v5.0
iSALUS	OfficeEMR™
Kryptiq	Providing connectivity for GE Centricity® EMR eScript Messenger v1.1
LighthouseMD	CareTracker v5.7
LSS Data Systems	Medical and Practice Management Suite Client Server v 5.54

(continues)

TABLE 7-1 *(Continued)*

Company	*Product*
M.D. Web Solutions	AMCIS EMR v4.2AP.S
McKesson	Horizon Ambulatory Care™ v9.4.1
MedAppz	iSuite v3.5.000
MedComSoft	Record Version 2006/Ultimate Edition
MedConnect, Inc	MedConnect EHR v 1.0
Medent	MEDENT v17
Medi-EMR	Medi-EMR
Medical Communication Systems	mMD.net EMR v9.1
Medical Information Systems, Inc.	ChartMaker
MedicWare	MedicWare EMR v6.7
MediNotes	MediNotes EMR Version 5.2
MedNet System	emr4MD
MedPlexus	MedPlexus
MedPlus	Care360 Physician Portal v5.0
Misys	eScript Version 3.5
Misys	Misys EMR v 8.10.1
NaviMedix	NaviNet v1.0.0.88
Netsmart - InfoScriber	InfoScriber
NewCrop	NewCrop v6.1
NextGen®	NextGen EMR v5.5
Noteworthy	Noteworthy EHR v6.0
OA Systems	Rx Cure v1.0
Polaris – Epichart	EpiChart v5.0
Practice Partner	Practice Partner v9.2.1
Prematics	ScriptTone v2199
Prime Clinical Systems	Patient Chart Manager V. 5.3
Purkinje	CareSeries Version 2.0
RelayHealth	eScript™ v7.2
RxNT	RxNT v 6.1.3
RxNT	EMR LITE v 7.0
SOAPware	SOAPware v5.0
SSIMED	EMRge™ v6.0.57
SynaMed	SynaMed v4.0.040423
VipaHealth Solutions	SmartEMR v5.5
Waiting Room Solutions	Web Based EMR & Practice Management System v3.0
Wellogic	Consult v3.10.4
ZixCorp	PocketScript v6.7

Source: SureScripts. *Choosing an EMR/Electronic Prescribing Application that is Right for Your Practice.* Available at: http://www.surescripts.com/pdf/BuyersGuide_Feb08Final-1.pdf. Accessed June 14, 2008. Reprinted with permission.

The below categories and features/functions are adapted from the SureScripts buyer's guide and are reprinted with permission.[7]

- Regulatory compliance: Does the solution comply with NCPDP Script standard (i.e., is it enabled for two-way communication with pharmacies through a connection to the Pharmacy Health Information Exchange or just one-way fax transmission of new prescription information)?
- Functionality: Can the vendor provide the following features?
  - Refill authorizations: Will the solution enable physicians or staff to receive refill requests from pharmacies directly on a computer instead of by fax or phone and send back approvals or denials electronically with minimal key strokes?
  - New prescriptions: Can new prescriptions be sent directly to the pharmacist's computer through a PDA, Desktop, Laptop, or Tablet PC instead of to their fax machine?
  - Rx history: Does the solution have the ability to be populated with patient medication histories from community pharmacies across providers?
  - User tools (i.e., chart labels, identifiers): Does the solution provide aids such as favorites-list or chart-labels to aid system use and practice workflow?
  - Drug-interaction checking: Does the solution provide alerts for drug to drug, drug to allergy or other checks for patient safety?
  - Formulary management: Does the solution display formulary information related to patient's drug coverage to help manage patient cost? Does it include all of the drugs available on a formulary or only the preferred formulary drugs?
- EMR solutions
  - Modules
    - Laboratory results
    - Charge captures
  - Modular EHR
    - Comprehensive medical record: Does the solution provide a comprehensive EHR that can be implemented in stages beginning with prescribing?

- Hardware
  - Mobile: Can the system be run through a PDA? Can peripherals be synchronized via a cradle or via Bluetooth options?
  - Desktop: Is an Internet connection all that is required, or does the system require specific software?
  - Remote computing: Does the solution provide access when prescribers are away from the office?
- Services
  - Training
  - Ongoing support 24/7
  - System interfaces: Can demographics for patients be loaded into the system effortlessly?
  - Updates: What is the process for obtaining updates?
- Costs
  - Hardware, software, and applicable services: What are the costs for all recommended hardware including any networking equipment?
  - Software and services: What are the one-time and ongoing costs for the software and any training and interfacing services?
  - Rebates, free trials, and other discounts: Are there any special offers such as free trials, rebates, or discounts?

Summary

This chapter has provided some issues that need to be considered when entering the e-prescribing milieu. The basics of e-prescribing have been presented using the SureScripts and RxHub companies as examples of connectivity between physicians and pharmacies (SureScripts) and between pharmacies and PBM companies (RxHub). The various features and functions that are a part of vendor systems were listed, and a descriptor of the features of the RxHub system was presented.

References

1. Hale P. *Electronic Prescribing Update* (HIMSS Fact Sheet). Available at: http://www.himss.org/content/files/CBO/Meeting7/ElectronicPrescribingUpdate.pdf. Accessed December 4, 2007.

2. RxHub National Patient Health Information Network. *RxHub Homepage*. Available at: http://www.rxhub.com. Accessed June 13, 2008.

3. RxHub National Patient Health Information Network. *RxHub PRN Patient Eligibility, Formulary & Benefits, and Medication History*. Available at: http://www.rxhub.com/index.php?option=com_content&task=view&id=31&Itemid=42. Accessed June 13, 2008.

4. RxHub National Patient Health Information Network. *RxHub SIG Electronic Prescription Connectivity to Pharmacy*. Available at: http://www.rxhub.com/index.php?option=com_content&task=view&id=32&Itemid=43. Accessed June 13, 2008.

5. RxHub National Patient Health Information Network. *RxHub MEDS™ Patient Medication History for Hospitals*. Available at: http://www.rxhub.com/index.php?option=com_content&task=view&id=33&Itemid=44. Accessed June 13, 2008.

6. RxHub National Patient Health Information Network. *RxHub Integration Services*. Available at: http://www.rxhub.net/index.php?option=com_content&task=view&id=34&Itemid=45. Accessed June 13, 2008.

7. SureScripts. *Choosing an EMR/Electronic Prescribing Application that is Right for Your Practice*. Available at: http://www.rxsuccess.com/best-practices.aspx?nav-resources. Accessed June 14, 2008.

EIGHT

The Impact of e-Prescribing on Pharmacists

Introduction

The profession of pharmacy potentially has the most to gain from widespread implementation of e-prescribing. The potential to use e-prescribing in medication therapy management service (MTMS) programs to help patients be more compliant, avoid adverse drug effects, and avoid therapeutic drug duplications and to monitor therapeutic outcomes will all be positive features of e-prescribing systems.

The uptake of e-prescribing technology has been sporadic as well as paradoxically controversial in some corners of the community pharmacy. In many cases, the community pharmacy response to such technological advances is passive rather than active and/or proactive response. For example, the disparity in application of e-prescribing within the community pharmacy is stark indeed. This is not an optional technology in my view; if laggard pharmacists do not embrace this technology, they will be left out.

e-Prescribing Uptake and Use by Community Pharmacy

There has been a difference in uptake of e-prescribing capabilities and readiness in the pharmacy community. For example, between 100% in the chain community and 20% in the independent community pharmacy have e-prescribing capabilities (please see Appendix C). These data have been suggested to be higher in the Sure-Scripts[r] *National Progress Report on e-Prescribing.*[1] In this referenced report, it is estimated that in 2007, a total of 40,000 community pharmacies were e-prescribing pharmacies. These pharmacies were classified as being 86% chain community pharmacies and 15% independent community pharmacies.[1] The report estimated that the number of pharmacies would increase to roughly 45,000 in 2008. Sure-Scripts estimated that in 2008 a total of 85,000 prescribers (95% of whom are physicians) would be e-prescribers. In 2007, during the first 10 months of the year, more e-prescribing activity occurred than that which was seen in the combined totals for the years 2004, 2005, and 2006![1] One of the major drivers in this increase has been attributed to the efforts of the software community pushing technology from faxed base to an electronically transferred base. The 10 highest e-prescribing states are listed in **Table 8-1**,[1] and the 10 least e-prescribing states are listed in **Table 8-2**.[1] These data are derived from examining the number of

TABLE 8-1 **Ranking of States with the Highest Percentage of e-Prescribed Prescriptions**

1. Massachusetts	6. Michigan
2. Rhode Island	7. North Carolina
3. Nevada	8. New Jersey
4. Delaware	9. Ohio
5. Maryland	10. Washington

Source: SureScripts. *National Progress Report on e-Prescribing.* Washington, DC: Author; December 2007. Available at: http://www.surescripts.com/pdf/National-Progress-Report-on-EPrescribing.pdf. Accessed June 17, 2008.

TABLE 8-2 **States* with the Lowest Percentage of e-Prescribed Prescriptions**

Alaska	Nebraska
Georgia	North Dakota
Hawaii	South Carolina
Iowa	South Dakota
Mississippi	Wisconsin

*This is not in any particular order of ranking; it is an alphabetized listing.
Source: SureScripts. *National Progress Report on e-Prescribing.* Washington, DC: Author; December 2007. Available at: http://www.surescripts.com/pdf/National-Progress-Report-on-EPrescribing.pdf. Accessed June 17, 2008.

actual e-prescribing prescriptions divided by the total number of eligible prescriptions that could have been e-prescribed.

States and e-Prescribing Status

From a percentage of 50% of the states allowing e-prescribing in 2004 to the current 100% enabling regulatory milieu climate, e-prescribing has been accepted and approved by each of the 50 states. The first transmission of an e-prescription on January 17, 2007, was made through the SureScripts network from a physician in the Washington, DC, area to a Rite Aid Pharmacy. Alaska was the final state to allow approval for e-prescribing. Many states and the federal government have played key roles in encouraging e-prescribing, with the hope for gain of fewer adverse effects and drug misadventures and an increase in quality of care. States gained esteem and visibility from the federal government and other experts as the best way to advance health IT efforts. As an example, Minnesota is the first state in the nation to require physicians contracting with the state employee health plan's medical networks to use e-prescribing by 2011.

Who Shall Pay?

There has been contentious debate about who will pay for e-prescribing segments. According to the Centers for Medicare and Medicaid Services (please see Appendix C):

> because e-prescribing is voluntary for pharmacies, dispensers who do not currently conduct e-prescribing would not incur any costs related to any of the provisions of this rule. However, we recognize that costs would be incurred by those dispensers that currently conduct e-prescribing transactions, as well as those who voluntarily implement e-prescribing during the period reflected in our regulatory impact analysis. Industry estimates are that close to 100 percent of the nation's retail chain pharmacies are connected live to an e-prescribing network, with over 95 percent of those connected to networks capable of receiving and exchanging formulary and benefit and medication history data. This is in contrast to only 20 percent of independent pharmacies that are connected to e-prescribing networks.

[Author's Note: Please see the introductory section above for differing data.]

Laborsky, writing about e-prescribing, asks: "Is this yet another situation where pharmacists unwillingly will bear the expense of this very much needed technology?"[2] Laborsky goes on to list five benefits of e-prescribing, while challenging the premise of these items:[2]

1. improved efficiency. (But with a cost to dispensing disparity as it exists today you cannot make up that disparity by increasing your volume with this technology.)
2. you can regain control of your business and profession . . . Does this really need a comment or should we just allow for the laughter to die down?
3. increased safety . . . Amen, they make a good point here . . . No more guessing, no more holding the Rx sideways above a light to decipher the M.D.'s writing.
4. less time consumed with getting the patient the formulary-approved drugs and less time in getting renewals that come over the electronic platform . . . I agree with the first point but not the second—patients will call you with the refill request, not the M.D.
5. more time to devote to patient care and running your business . . . You will have more time, but not for patients and your business, but more time to fill more prescriptions for less money.

The cost per prescription for e-prescribed prescriptions is estimated to be between 21.5¢ and 50¢. Cost savings accruing to the payers have been estimated to be between 75¢ and $3.20 per prescription. According to the New Mexico Prescription Improvement Coalition, the time savings and associated reduction in pharmacy costs is estimated to be 97¢ for new prescriptions and 37¢ for refill prescriptions.[3]

Pharmacist Criticism

A pharmacist from Pflugerville, Texas, responding to the request for postings to the Labrosky posting, states:[2]

It has been my experience thus far that the chance of errors in prescribing is much greater with electronic prescribing than traditional methods. Those who tout e-prescribing as safer obviously haven't worked much in a pharmacy to observe thy system in actual practice. Their interests are self serving in trying to sell technology for the sake of technology and their profits, without any practical advantages whatsoever. It is so much easier to erroneously click on the wrong button than to write out the wrong drug. I have spent much more time contacting the doctors in the past several months to clarify electronic prescriptions (wrong drug, strength, directions) than I have in the last several years with traditional prescriptions.

So, there are real questions about financing e-prescribing and who the ultimate payer will be. Whether the charges accruing to pharmacies will be an all-inclusive monthly fee, a pay per transaction fee, or a combination of both will remain to be seen. It is conceivable that those unwilling to set in place e-prescribing technologies in their pharmacies may see prescription volumes drop precipitously.

Increasing Volume of Prescriptions

In a 19-month study completed by Walgreen Company, pharmacists saw better than an 11% increase in the number of prescriptions at pharmacies during the study period.[4] The study followed a before-and-after analysis of the effect of e-prescribing on prescription volume. Aiding Walgreen in the study were the e-prescribing exchange SureScripts and data-miner IMS Health.[4] One data point that can be derived from analyzing the e-prescribing patterns is the number of prescriptions that are originated by physicians or other prescribers that are not initially picked up by patients.

Enhanced Professional Role

Pharmacists in a study carried out in the United Kingdom felt that they would have more of a professional role with the implementation of e-prescribing.[5] Part of this sentiment was driven by the view that community pharmacists would have greater involvement in medicines management, particularly for chronic conditions.[5] Both general practitioners and pharmacists concurred on this benefit of e-prescribing. Turf issues that affect so much of the delivery of health care do not seem to be impediments at this point to the adoption of e-prescribing not only in the United States but elsewhere.

e-Prescriptions and the Identification of Drug Interactions Highlighting the Role of Pharmacists

One means of enhancing the pharmacist's role is through identification of drug interactions by e-prescribing systems. The subsequent avoidance of further medical problems due to these alerts is crucial. An example Bodine provides of the difference e-prescribing can make involves the Southeast Michigan e-Prescribing Initiative.[6] When the Henry Ford Medical Group signed on, its 600 participating physicians wrote more than 1 million e-prescriptions within 18 months. Of those prescriptions, more than 98,000 were changed or cancelled due to drug-drug interaction alerts (a rate of 9.8%), and more than 63,000 were changed or cancelled because of formulary alerts. This medical group expected to save more than $1 million per year by using e-prescribing.[6]

In addition to pharmacy alerts and actions by the pharmacists, these systems can alert physicians to potential interactions before orders are processed. Therefore, the impact may be greater as a whole than only examining the pharmacist/physician's actions alone.

The Benefit of Far Fewer Phone Calls

e-Prescribing does offer the tantalizing time-saving aspect of fewer phone calls necessary to clarify prescriptions, formularies, eligibility, and other issues. It is seriously doubtful that the need to phone PBMs, other third-party program administrators, physicians, and/or patients will be completely eliminated, but there will be serious reductions in the need for such and would thus allow pharmacists conceivably much more time to spend on clinical functions. Estimates place the economic costs of callbacks for physicians' practices to be between $5 and $7 per prescription.

It has been estimated that there are over 3.3 billion prescriptions written in the United States yearly. In addition, there are many deaths that have been suggested to be a result of pharmacists' inability to correctly interpret physicians' wishes from written prescriptions. Estimates suggest that 1.5 million mistakes in prescription discernment can be impacted by e-prescribing technologies.

e-Prescribing for Controlled Substances

Attempts have been made to control misuse of the Drug Enforcement Administration (DEA) Scheduled drugs (Schedules II, III, IV, V) since the mid-1960s.

There have been attempts to reign in inappropriate use of these Scheduled drugs via law enforcement, medical, and pharmacy impacts. Most recently, there have been requirements for Scheduled drugs to be written on a triplicate prescription pad for governmental programs such as Medicaid. The state of New York has also had triplicate prescriptions required for some time for controlled substances. Many feel that e-prescribing will enable a more successful approach to misuse of Scheduled drugs by patients.

CMS and e-Prescribing and Pharmacists

The CMS has placed a Notice of Proposed Rule Making on display at the Federal Register announcing a proposal to adopt the Formulary and Benefits and Medication History e-prescribing standards for the prescription drug program. The proposed rule is listed in its entirety in Appendix D. The rule also calls for industry comments on several matters, including the feasibility of adopting a standard for fill status.

The CMS standard for formulary and benefits allows prescribers to see up front which drugs are covered under a beneficiary's Medicare drug benefit plan as well as a list of alternative drugs.[7] This functionality improves compliance, reduces administrative overhead for doctors and pharmacists, and allows the provider in many cases to substitute a generic drug, thus saving the patient money. With medication history, providers will know at the point of care which drugs have been prescribed and claimed by their patients and which drugs could have harmful interactions. CMS has undertaken pilot studies for which the results can be found at the following link: http://www.cms.hhs.gov/EPrescribing/Downloads/E-RxReporttoCongress.pdf.[7]

While e-prescribing is voluntary under the Medicare prescription drug benefit, providers and pharmacies that electronically transmit prescriptions for Medicare covered drugs are required to comply with any applicable final standards that are in effect. Further, all Part D plans are required to maintain e-prescribing systems that conform to the final standards.[7] CMS has asked for comments on the proposed rule.

U.S. Department of Health and Human Services Report

In a recently released report to Congress, HHS secretary Michael Leavitt announced the results of an e-prescribing pilot project that support the adoption of new e-prescribing standards.[7] These standards, required by the Medicare Modernization Act of 2003, would help cut both medication errors and health care costs.

Leavitt noted:[8(p.1)]

Electronic prescribing improves efficiencies while helping to eliminate potentially harmful drug interactions and other medication problems. It also solves the problem of hard-to-read handwritten prescriptions. Additionally, such health information technologies promote affordability by allowing physicians to know which medications are covered by their patients' Part D plans.

The pilot project demonstrated that 3 initial standards are already capable of supporting e-prescribing transactions in Medicare Part D. These are standard transactions that provide physicians with patients' formulary and benefit information, medication history, and the fill status of their medications.[8(p.1)]

Leavitt went on to posit: "The findings in this report, along with previously adopted foundation standards, demonstrate that HHS is effectively advancing electronic prescribing which will continue to help Medicare beneficiaries receive higher quality care."[8(p.1)]

The report also found that, with some adjustments, e-prescribing can work successfully in long-term care settings. Some of the initial e-prescribing standards tested by the pilot project were found to have potential but still need further development if they are to be adopted as e-prescribing standards. These include standards used to convey structured patient instructions, a terminology to describe clinical drugs, and messages that convey prior authorization information.[8]

The pilot project, conducted through an interagency agreement between CMS and the Agency for Healthcare Research and Quality (AHRQ), selected 5 pilot sites operating in 8 states to test initial standards to determine if they were ready for widespread adoption. Those pilot sites were Achieve Healthcare Information Technologies, LLP, Eden Prairie, Minnesota; Brigham and Women's Hospital, Boston, Massachusetts; Rand Corporation, Santa Monica, California; SureScripts, LLC, Alexandria, Virginia; and University Hospitals Health System, Cleveland, Ohio.[9]

Conclusions from the National Opinion Research Center

The following is an evaluation conducted by the National Opinion Research Center (NORC) regarding the effects on pharmacies and pharmacists at their 5 e-prescribing pilot study sites:[9(p.67–68)]

> The main finding of all the sites is that the role of surrogates—surrogates include nurse practitioners, physician assistants, physician office staff (nurses [registered nurses, licensed practical nurses, or licensed vocational nurses], or office clerical personnel), etc., was underappreciated in prescribing workflow generally, and particularly post e-prescribing adoption. In the paper-based prescribing era, many medications were called into pharmacies without physician intervention. In the e-prescribing era, where e-prescribing can eliminate phone time and cost, the same office-based personnel now take on a larger role. Although this improves office efficiency, the impact on patient safety is not established.
>
> One project site (Achieve) noted that this workflow might compromise the attention given to drug allergy alerts. This phenomenon deserves additional study and should become a part of the education provided to e-prescribing physicians.
>
> Another important finding from these groups is that in almost no setting did e-prescribing replace the need for paper-based prescribing. Factors important in this observation include the inability to manage future orders electronically, the inability to submit Schedule II controlled substance prescriptions using the SCRIPT standards, and the time pressures that prescribers feel. The impact of this finding on workflow is seen in the highly variable use of e-prescribing features.
>
> One of the sites with the strongest study design for assessing workflow change reported notable reductions in workflow as a result of e-prescribing. However, in those groups with pre-existing electronic health records or e-prescribing, workflow transformation might have occurred before the beginning of the study and would also not likely be found. Additional longitudinal studies will be needed to explore this question in more depth.
>
> Implementation of e-prescribing had the potential to dramatically change pharmacy workflow, in several cases with negative consequences.

For example, two sites mentioned that pharmacies were unable to transfer received SCRIPT messages to their pharmacy system. Patient concerns almost always included challenges at the pharmacy related to pharmacy workflow of electronically submitted new prescriptions. In short, additional studies of outpatient pharmacies, with communication to pharmacy information systems vendors are needed.

In analyses, particularly those by Ohio KePRO/UHMP, pilot sites identified a shift from phone-based to e-prescribing based refill and renewal prescriptions. Based on the provider practice surveys, the new e-prescribing workflows for refills and renewals may generate efficiencies for small physician offices. In addition, these findings suggest that in the current form, e-prescribing tools may decrease the reliance on verbal orders and phone transmission of those orders. However, the use of surrogates may be associated with a concomitant increase in "verbal orders"—none of the sites have clearly outlined how providers are involved in the cognitive aspects of prescribing when surrogates act as their agents.

HHS Projections for e-Prescribing Benefits Emanating from the Pilot Projects

Johnston et al have suggested that e-prescribing could avoid more than 2 million adverse drug events annually, and—of this number—an estimated 130,000 that could be life-threatening.[10] Even so, 5 government-funded e-prescribing pilot projects did not establish the effect on patient safety noting the role of office staff members in handling e-prescribing tasks.[9] The study report concluded that the effect on safety requires more study.[9]

e-Prescribing Pilot Showed Technology Benefits

The report contains a great deal of information that may help the e-prescribing industry pursue its mission to make e-prescribing connectivity the standard of practice throughout the country.[9] In brief, the pilots assessed the functionality and readiness to implement e-prescribing. Findings from the report include the following:[9]

- Three technical standards for medication history, formulary and benefits, and prescription fill status notification are ready to be implemented as part of the Medicare Part D drug benefit plan. (These 3 standards are in production with SureScripts Pharmacy Health Information Exchange.)

- Standards for structured and codified SIG, RxNorm, and prior authorization were unable to convey the information needed for use in Medicare Part D in their current state.

- The grantees/contractor tracked various outcomes of e-prescribing with the following findings:
  - Workflow: Workflow improves for both prescribers and pharmacists with direct computer to computer transmission and improved connectivity to e-prescribing networks and communication with outside entities.
  - Prescriber utilization of e-prescribing: Office staff plays a significant role in e-prescribing, particularly in the long-term care setting.
  - Physician uptake: Adoption rates/retention were reasonable and, barring technical problems related to electronic devices and incomplete patient data, retention was generally good.
  - Patient satisfaction: There was limited pilot site experience in this area, but of the small sample surveyed, adults under 65 years of age preferred e-prescribing over paper.
  - Formulary vs. generic prescribing: The role of e-prescribing in the use of formulary medication and generics is still very preliminary, with prescribers uncertain about the accuracy and completeness of formulary information.
  - Medication history utilization: Providers may have been unaware of this function's availability; comments ranged from a perception of inaccurate medication histories to it being a good supplement to patient self-reporting.

Changes in Number of Callbacks from Pharmacy to Prescribers

Almost 30% of prescriptions require pharmacy callbacks, resulting in 900 million prescription-related telephone calls annually.[7] Many of these calls are for issues that should not arise in a well-implemented e-prescribing system, such as clarification of handwriting or renewal requests.

NORC Summary and Conclusions

The findings from the NORC study conducted on behalf of AHRQ are instructive for the eventual widespread use of e-prescribing.[10(p.67)]

Collection of data about callbacks is difficult, as these pilots discovered. However, it appears that e-prescribing may represent a component of cost-shifting—providing more efficiency in practice settings, but with unknown and possible deleterious effects at the dispensing end of the continuum. More studies need to be done to evaluate this phenomenon, given both the data about the rarity of true "end-to-end" e-prescribing, and the theme of negative impact on the workflow of pharmacists at this transition point.

Time Savings
The findings from the NORC study conducted on behalf of AHRQ provide data on time savings accruing for pharmacy staff due to e-prescribing. The NORC study concludes:[10(p.61)]

Further analysis was conducted to determine the effect of number of medications for time spent for the above mentioned tasks. Time spent on task was significantly associated with number of medications in a positive direction indicating that as the number of medication increases so does the time spent on the task (except for the task of insurance rejections). Yet there was no evidence to suggest that the e-prescribing system has any impact on the relationship that exists between number of medication and time spent on a task.

Summary

Pharmacists have much to gain from embracing e-prescribing. Tangible benefits may include an increase in prescription volume, an enhanced professional role recognized by both physicians and pharmacists, an ability to reduce drug errors due to illegible handwriting on traditional prescriptions written by prescribers, a reduction of adverse drug events, a better handle on reducing Scheduled drug abuse and patient abuse through "doctor and/or pharmacy shopping," and a chance to play an ever more important and necessary role in the evolution of health IT conception, structure, implementation, and applications.

Much can be lost as well by not participating as a full partner in e-prescribing platforms, applications, and implementations. There will be a segment of pharmacy that will embrace this technology and has already. If a broader representation of pharmacy does not begin to view health IT, e-prescribing, and EHR in a proactive and active participatory fashion, a significant segment of the pharmacy community will be left behind. The opportunity to then catch up with colleagues or early adopters may not be reemerging for later participation consideration.

References

1. SureScripts. *National Progress Report on e-Prescribing.* Washington, DC: Author; December 2007. Available at: http://www.surescripts.com/pdf/National-Progress-Report-on-EPrescribing.pdf. Accessed June 17, 2008.
2. Laborsky J. *Drug Topics Publisher's Blog: e-Prescribing—Pharmacy Pays to Play.* Available at: http://www.drugtopics.com/drugtopics/Publisher's+Blog/Publishers-Blog-E-prescribing151pharmacy-pays-to-p/ArticleStandard/Article/detail/457191?contextCategory Id=42266. Accessed January 3, 2008.
3. New Mexico Prescription Improvement Coalition. *NMMRA Homepage.* Available at: http://www.nmmra.org. Accessed June 13, 2008.
4. Conn J. e-Prescribing ups number of prescriptions filled. *Mod Healthcare.* October 16, 2007;Online. Available at: http://modernhealthcare.com/apps/pbcs.dll/article?AID=/20071016/FREE/71016001. Accessed January 3, 2008.
5. Porteous T, Bond C, Robertson R, Hannaford P, Reiter E. Electronic transfer of prescription-related information: comparing views of patients, general practitioners, and pharmacists. *Br J Gen Pract.* 2003;53:204–209.
6. Bodine WK. e-Prescribing can make a difference for Medicare Part D. *Pharm Times.* April 2007. Available at: http://www.pharmacytimes.com/issues/articles/2007-04_4600.asp. Accessed March 7, 2008.
7. Leavitt MO. *Pilot Testing of Initial Electronic Prescribing Standards—Cooperative Agreements Required Under Section 1860D-(4) (e) of the Social Security Act as Amended by the Medicare Prescription Drug, Improvement, and Modernization Action (MMA) of 2003.* Available at: http://www.cms.hhs.gov/EPrescribing. Accessed November 24, 2007.
8. U.S. Department of Health and Human Services. *HHS Issues Report to Congress on e-Prescribing: Electronic Prescribing to Cut Errors and Costs* [News Release April 17, 2007]. Available at: http://www.hhs.gov/news/press/2007pres/04/20070417e.html. Accessed June 13, 2008.
9. The National Opinion Research Center (NORC) at the University of Chicago. *Findings from the Evaluation of e-Prescribing Pilot Sites* [AHRQ Publication No. 07-0047-EF]. Chicago: Author; April 2007.
10. Johnston D, Pan E, Middleton B, Walker J, Bates DW. *The Value of Computerized Order Entry in Ambulatory Settings.* Boston: Center for Information Technology Leadership; 2004.

NINE

The Impact of e-Prescribing on Physicians

Introduction

It is not an overstatement to say that the success of e-prescribing both short term and long term is dependent upon physician acceptance and continued utilization. All systems can be in place for use and access, but the key profession in e-prescribing is medicine. Current physician e-prescribing rates have been low, but, as is the case with any new technology rates, they will increase as e-prescribing become ubiquitous. Rates have been less than 10% across the country; more about these data later.

Studies indicate that much remains to be accomplished before widespread physician acceptance and the ultimate utilization of e-prescribing. For example, findings from a qualitative study of physician practices suggest that substantial gaps may exist between advocates' vision of e-prescribing and how physicians use commercial e-prescribing systems today.[1] Grossman et al note:[1(p.w393)]

> While physicians were positive about the most basic e-prescribing features, they reported major barriers to maintaining complete patient medication lists, using clinical decision support, obtaining formulary data, and electronically transmitting prescriptions to pharmacies. Three factors

help explain the gaps: product limitations, external implementation challenges, and physicians' preferences about using specific product features.

A realistic alignment of advocates' promotion and assessment and physician acceptance must be accomplished before e-prescribing can reach its promised potential. Physicians in the United Kingdom have expressed concerns about the security of EMRs and associated features (i.e., e-prescribing).[2] The poll was carried out online over Christmas 2007. In general, the general practitioners (GPs), who have the greater experience of IT systems, are more skeptical than the consultants. In the poll, physicians were asked the question: "Do the benefits of electronic patient records outweigh the risks?" A narrow majority of all doctors polled said no. Among GPs, the gap was much wider, with almost two-thirds doubting that the benefits would outweigh the risks.[2]

The promise of a reduction in physicians' administrative expenses due to enhanced legibility of prescriptions and time-saving features of electronic processing of refills remains great. However, implementation challenges include the following:

- The need for a critical mass of pharmacies to participate: Unless a far greater percentage of pharmacies are enabled to receive e-prescriptions, the promise of future time and error savings will not be readily fulfilled.

- The need for adequate software installation for physicians' use: Physicians need to have appropriate software for transmission of e-prescriptions; furthermore, the key to success for software installation and application is a transparent realization of successful interoperability between systems.

- A need for a critical mass of medical history data that is secure and accessible.

Benefits for Physicians

e-Prescribing holds great promise to enhance the quality of care provided by physicians. The number of e-prescribing physicians will need to significantly increase for widespread enhancement of quality of care.[3] In a summary report on e-prescribing, Kilbridge notes the benefits that can be realized by physicians with e-prescribing.[4] He suggests the greatest benefit to physicians comes from enhanced efficiencies due to:[4]

- A reduction in the number of callbacks to and from pharmacies to clarify certain prescription components
- Illegible prescriptions
- Nonformulary medications
- Potential drug interactions
- Incorrect dosages
- Refill requests

In 2001, in an assessment of the impact of callbacks to and from physicians to pharmacies, Versel estimated that there were 150 million calls a year from pharmacies to physicians to clarify prescription orders.[5] Kilbridge suggests that increased patient satisfaction with physician care will also be a tangible result of e-prescribing and the benefits derived from the technology.[4]

Who Shall Pay?

The CMS presents "who shall pay" information in the e-prescribing final rule at 70-FR-67589, the estimated start-up costs for e-prescribing for providers and/or dispensers. Based on industry input, we cited approximately $3,000 for annual support, maintenance, infrastructure, and licensing costs. Physicians at that time reported paying user-based licensing fees ranging from $80 to $400 per month. (Please see Appendix D for this CMS-proposed rule.) It has been noted that physicians with slower practices have been loath to invest significant sums to set in place e-prescribing systems.[4] However, I feel that in future e-prescribing milieus, physicians will be provided such systems free of charge. This is in no small part due to the enhancement of quality and accuracy in prescribing that accrues due to e-prescribing applications. These cost-free platforms will include those that can be adapted for handheld devices, such as PDAs.

Enhanced Patient Compliance

Fincham has suggested that compliance estimates on behalf of patients should be considered for inclusion in "vital signs" sections of medical records, electronic or otherwise.[6] These compliance estimates can be viewed as just as important as the other crucial measures that are included in assessing patients. Blood pressure measurements are merely isolated determinations if no concomitant assessments and recordings of adherence to treatment regimens for hypertension are also made. Pulse values for a congestive heart failure patient are of little use if compliance with treatments is not also assessed at the same time. One cannot hide values for weight, height, temperature, blood pressure, or pulse readings when having vital signs evaluated and recorded. In the same vein, patients need to feel comfortable having compliance estimates gleaned and recorded in patient medical records. This may require multiple entries for multiple drugs taken, and can be time consuming but can be easily accomplished with e-prescribing associated accoutrements. But, it would appear to be a very good use of time and energy.

Assuming patients are compliant when they actually are not and therefore failing to provide additional, individualized compliance aids or further pharmacotherapy that might be easier complied with is ultimately more time consuming and vastly more costly for all involved.[6] It is not uncommon for physicians to assume patients are compliant with therapies; this is especially so if physicians are not apprised of noncompliance either by the patient and/or pharmacist.

Menu-Driven Features Enhancing Prescribing Accuracy

Many of the e-prescribing platforms house programs that will simplify physicians' prescribing activities and enhance the quality of prescribing for them. Some of these enhancements include the following:

- Avoidance of duplicate prescriptions that may be written by other physicians from whom patients seek care (This presupposes that all physicians writing prescriptions for specific patients are e-prescribing and are able to access drug profiles for the specific patients in question.)
- Detection of drug-drug and/or drug-laboratory interactions
- Detection of drug allergies through alerts
- Accuracy of drug diagnosis(es)
- Increased dosing accuracy for seniors, pediatric, or immunocompromised patients

Quality of Care Enhancement

Physicians are currently incentivized in various programs for enhancing quality of care. Such pay-for-performance (P4P) programs include segments rewarding physicians for achieving successful patient outcomes in the populations they serve. Enhancing the successful outcomes via e-prescribing will no doubt be segments of such P4P programs in the future. These outcomes may be error reduction, enhanced compliance, avoidance of drug interactions, and/or eliminating erroneous prescriptions for the wrong patient or wrong dose or nonformulary drug selections.

The Benefit of Far Fewer Phone Calls

e-Prescribing does offer the tantalizing, time-saving aspect of fewer phone calls necessary to clarify prescriptions, formularies, eligibility, and the like. It is seriously doubtful that the need to phone PBMs, other third-party program administrators, physicians, and/or patients will be eliminated, but there will be serious reductions in the need for such and would thus allow pharmacists conceivably much more time to spend on clinical functions.

It has been estimated that there are over 3.3 billion prescriptions written in the United States yearly. There are many deaths that have been suggested to be a result of pharmacists' inability to correctly interpret physicians' wishes from written prescriptions. Estimates suggest that 1.5 million mistakes in prescription discernment can be impacted by e-prescribing technologies.

e-Prescribing for Controlled Substances

There have been attempts to control misuse of the Drug Enforcement Administration (DEA) Scheduled drugs (Schedules II, III, IV, V) since the mid-1960s. There have been attempts to reign in inappropriate use of these Scheduled drugs via law enforcement, medical, and pharmacy impacts. Most recently, there have been requirements for Scheduled drugs to be written on a triplicate prescription pad for governmental programs such as Medicaid. The state of New York also has had triplicate prescriptions required for some time for controlled substances. Many feel that e-prescribing will enable a more successful approach to misuse of Scheduled drugs by patients; however, at present this is not allowed.

e-Prescribing Pilot Showed Technology Benefits

As noted in Chapter 8, e-prescribing pilot studies have been instructive in pointing out the many benefits of e-prescribing. In brief, the pilots assessed the functionality and readiness to implement e-prescribing. Findings from the report include the following:[7]

- Three technical standards for medication history, formulary and benefits, and prescription fill status notification are ready to be implemented as part of the Medicare Part D drug benefit plan. (These 3 standards are in production with SureScripts Pharmacy Health Information Exchange.)

- Standards for structured and codified SIG, RxNorm, and prior authorization were unable to convey the information needed for use in Medicare Part D in their current state.

- The grantees/contractor tracked various outcomes of e-prescribing with the following findings:
  - Workflow: Workflow improves for both prescribers and pharmacists with direct computer to computer transmission and improved connectivity to e-prescribing networks and communication with outside entities.
  - Prescriber utilization of e-prescribing: Office staff plays a significant role in e-prescribing, particularly in the long-term care setting.
  - Physician uptake: Adoption rates/retention were reasonable and, barring technical problems related to electronic devices and incomplete patient data, retention was generally good.
  - Patient satisfaction: There was limited pilot site experience in this area, but of the small sample surveyed, adults under 65 years of age preferred e-prescribing over paper.
  - Formulary vs. generic prescribing: The role of e-prescribing in the use of formulary medication and generics is still very preliminary, with prescribers uncertain about the accuracy and completeness of formulary information.
  - Medication history utilization: Providers may have been unaware of this function's availability; comments ranged from a perception of inaccurate medication histories to it being a good supplement to patient self-reporting.

Disadvantages for Physicians

The disadvantages for physicians in using e-prescribing as a method to "write" prescriptions are meager in scope and breadth and depth. (The term "write" for indicating how physicians and prescribers transmit prescriptions becomes archaic when considering the widespread application of e-prescribing!) Any of the following disadvantages will be diminished as more and more physicians and other prescribers begin to and continue to utilize e-prescribing in the near and long term.

Lack of Use at Present

Estimates of the number of e-prescribed prescriptions in 2007 reached 35 million and are projected to be 100 million in 2008.[3] (These data include both new and refill prescription orders.) Although this increase of 186% between 2007 and 2008 is noteworthy, the percentage of prescriptions e-prescribed is still low, estimated at 2% in 2007.[3] These data, regardless of how they are viewed, are not solely specific to physicians' actions—if pharmacies are not e-prescription-ready, physicians cannot e-prescribe!

Lack of Access to Certified Systems

A certified application provides physicians with an electronic connection to pharmacies and the instructions on how to go about making the connection. Many physicians are unaware that they have this capability in their systems, and as such, underutilize or do not utilize e-prescribing options. (Please see Table 7-1 for a listing of companies and products that are available for physicians to enable e-prescribing in their practices. This listing is updated as of June 2008; note that frequent additions and deletions are commonplace with this technology.)

Summary

The pilot tests of e-prescribing completed in 2007 provide a good assessment of the benefits of e-prescribing as they relate to physicians and other prescribers.[8] In the report, Leavitt points to the benefits accruing to physicians with adoption of e-prescribing in the 5 documented case studies.[8]

Findings from Outcomes Studies

Conclusions reached from the *Findings from the Evaluation of e-Prescribing Pilot Sites* conducted by the University of Chicago—The National Opinion Research Center (NORC) regarding effects on pharmacies and pharmacists within the 5 pilot study sites indicate a mixed conclusion for the at-present benefits of e-prescribing for physicians.[8]

The NORC study summarized the results from the 5 pilot studies as such:[8(p.10–11)]

> In addition to testing the functionality of e-prescribing standards, pilot sites tracked various outcomes of e-prescribing in their pilots. The following observations were made by the evaluation team:
>
> - Prescriber uptake and satisfaction: Adoption and retention of e-prescribing among providers was generally good. In order to facilitate prescriber adoption, the evaluation team recommends institutions implementing e-prescribing take into account the role of their organizational culture and prepare for possible "surrogate prescribing" (see below).
>
> - Prescriber and pharmacy workflow changes: One finding that was consistent across all sites was that prescribers' staff played a much more important role in the e-prescribing process than most pilot sites had anticipated. The evaluation team recommends that future e-prescribing efforts take the role of these staff, or "surrogate prescribers" into account in their planning. Another finding was that e-prescribing almost never replaced the need for paper-based prescribing, leading to highly variable use of e-prescribing features. In addition, implementation of e-prescribing can create dramatic "paradigm shifts" in pharmacy workflow. Pharmacies implementing e-prescribing, therefore, must allocate sufficient resources to deal with substantial change management. Finally, preliminary findings suggest that e-prescribing tools may decrease reliance on verbal orders and generate certain efficiencies for small physician offices. Proof of such efficiencies is still relatively preliminary, however.
>
> - Changes in number of callbacks from pharmacy to prescribers: Findings reported by some pilots suggest that e-prescribing reduces the number of phone time for physician practices while potentially decreasing efficiency on the pharmacy through an

increase in the number of callbacks required to complete a prescription. Yet other pilots found a decrease in callbacks related specifically to drug coverage issues. Given these inconsistencies, the evaluation team recommends that further study is required to acquire a more complete understanding of this potentially "cost-shifting" phenomenon.

- Patient satisfaction: According to surveys from one pilot site, most patients are satisfied with e-prescribing. Future studies should investigate further into patient perspectives to see what may cause dissatisfaction.

- Use of medication history functions: Overall, the pilots' findings demonstrated poor adoption of this functionality. We recommend further research to determine better ways for displaying and maintaining up-to-date medication histories to providers.

- Changes in prescription renewal and new prescription rates: The long term care site reported a reduction in new prescription rates, indicating the possibility that e-prescribing may reduce the tendency for such patients to accumulate unnecessary active medications.

- Inappropriate prescribing rates: The study period was too brief to make a measurable difference in the number of inappropriately prescribed medications.

- Medication errors, adverse drug events, hospitalizations and ED visit rates: The data on medication errors and ADEs is not conclusive and is in a preliminary state. The pilots will proceed with additional analysis to determine more precisely the impact of e-prescribing on patient safety.

- Use of on-formulary medications and generics: Clinicians surveyed by the pilots were concerned about the accuracy of formulary information provided by e-prescribing systems. Further studies will need to assess the perceived and actual quality of this information. In addition, generic prescribing that automatically allow for generic substitution may increase the rate of generic prescribing.

- Change in fill status rates: Fill status use was extremely limited due to the difficult implementation of this standard.

- Improved security and reliability of prescriptions: Only one of the sites investigated this issue; however, the security architecture they developed shows that the industry is taking important steps towards implementing systems that are secure and reliable. Future studies should test e-prescribing to ensure it meets security standards.

Pilot Testing of Initial e-Prescribing Standards

Finally, from the *Pilot Testing of Initial Electronic Prescribing Standards* report to Congress, Leavitt summarizes:[8(p.29–30)]

Electronic prescribing is still in its infancy. While the pilot sites have demonstrated the potential for effective standards-based implementation of three of the initial standards, there is additional work to be done on the three remaining initial standards in order to make them suitable for adoption for Part D. The testing of the initial standards conducted by the pilot project reflects each respective standard's technical ability to convey the needed information, but implementation issues remain. It is anticipated that these implementation issues will be addressed through industry and stakeholder input into the established process leading up to the issuance of final e-prescribing standards.

Additionally, the pilot project was impacted by the limited amount of time in which to recruit grantees/contractor and conduct pilot site activities; the small size of the pilot sites themselves which may or may not represent a statistically significant sample; and the ability of the grantees/contractor to recruit the right set of participants to make the outcomes meaningful.

The majority of practices consist in size of one to two physicians. Their adoption of e-prescribing may be slower. Their overall requirements for support will be higher than physicians in larger practices, who will likely deploy e-prescribing on the way toward more comprehensive, patient-focused health information technology systems.

On the surface, e-prescribing involves getting a prescription from point A to point B. In reality, the complexity of e-prescribing necessitates testing of all aspects of the process and determining which standards can support each of the steps in that process. The testing and adoption of this second layer of standards as demonstrated by the pilot sites should be just part of an ongoing effort to continue to work with industry, standards setting organizations and other interested stakeholders to fully adopt and implement electronic prescribing in order to reap its many potential benefits.

Final Word

As more follow-ups studies and summary reports are available, the continuing benefits of e-prescribing for physicians will become apparent, and the positive momentum will increase accordingly.

References

1. Grossman JM, Gerland A, Reed MC, et al. Physicians' experiences using commercial e-prescribing systems. *Health Aff*. 2007;Web exclusive:w393–w404.
2. Hawkes N. Four out of five doctors believe patient database will be at risk. *The Times*. December 31, 2007. Available at: http://www.timesonline.co.uk. Accessed January 7, 2008.
3. SureScripts. *National Progress Report on e-Prescribing*. Washington, DC: Author; December 2007.
4. Kilbridge P. *e-Prescribing*. Oakland CA: California HealthCare Foundation; 2001.
5. Versel N. Script central: PBMs create electronic hub to link pharmacies, physicians. *Mod Physician*. 2001;5(6):6.
6. Fincham JE. Pharmacists, patient drug use and misuse, and necessary evolving professional roles. *Harvard Health Pol Rev*. 2006;7(1):169–179.
7. The National Opinion Research Center (NORC) at the University of Chicago. *Findings from the Evaluation of e-Prescribing Pilot Sites* [AHRQ Publication No. 07-0047-EF]. Chicago: Author; April 2007.
8. Leavitt MO. *Pilot Testing of Initial Electronic Prescribing Standards—Cooperative Agreements Required Under Section 1860d-(4)(E) of the Social Security Act as Amended by the Medicare Prescription Drug, Improvement, and Modernization Action (MMA) of 2003*. Available at: http://www.cms.hhs.gov/EPrescribing. Accessed November 24, 2007.

TEN

The Impact of e-Prescribing on Patients

Introduction

The U.S. health care system has not been a patient-centered milieu for decades. There have been fundamental flaws in the drug use process in the United States. Medication compliance hovers around 50%, prescription drug misuse is rampant, OTC medications are misused, ADEs occur (many of which are preventable), antibiotic misuse has led to drug-resistant strains of many bacteria, and, despite recent changes to Medicare providing coverage for outpatient medications for many seniors, many other patients remain uninsured with respect to prescription medications. However, the positive effect of e-prescribing on patients holds the potential to be an enormous benefit for both patients and patient care. This revolutionary change in the ordering of prescription medications holds enormous possibilities to finally make the patient the center of health care delivery.

Drug Use Is Complex: e-Prescribing Can Help Simplify

The use of drugs as a form of medical treatment in the United States constitutes an enormously complex process. Individuals can purchase medications through numerous outlets. OTC medications can be purchased in pharmacies, in grocery stores, in supermarkets, in convenience stores, via the Internet, and through any number of additional venues. Prescriptions can be purchased through traditional channels (community chain and independent pharmacies, food market pharmacies), through mail service pharmacies, through the Internet, through physicians, through health care institutions, and elsewhere. e-Prescribing provides physicians, pharmacists, nurses, and most importantly, patients and their caregivers with a technology to better assess appropriateness, economic aspects, and outcomes with the use of prescription medications.

Problems with Monitoring Drug Use

Because of this proliferation of outlets for drug acquisition, the monitoring of the positive and negative outcomes of the use of these drugs (both prescription and OTC) can be disjointed and incomplete. So what are the current problems? Self-medication, wide array of purchasing options, and/or lack of insurance coverage are all problematic at present.

Self-Medication

Self-medication can be broadly defined as a decision made by a patient to consume a drug without the explicit approval or direction of a health professional. Self-medication increased dramatically in the late 20th century and continues on abated in the 21st century. Many contemporary developments have continued to fuel this increase. There are ever increasing locations from which to purchase OTC medications. There have been many medications switched to OTC classification from prescription-only classification in the last 50 years. In addition, patients are increasingly becoming comfortable with self-diagnosis and self-selection of OTC remedies. These changes may, in part, be fueled by direct marketing to consumers. Direct-to-consumer advertising for prescription drugs has doubled in the recent past, from $1.1 billion in 1997 to $2.7 billion in 2001.[1] As drugs have been switched from prescription to OTC status, the advertising and promotion of these drugs increase as well.

Where Drugs Are Obtained

Patients consume medications, herbal product, OTC medications and remedies, and social drugs (tobacco, alcoholic beverages, caffeine-containing beverages, or drugs of abuse) from numerous sources, often unbeknownst to health care providers.

These processes of obtaining medications, regardless of classification, will not be affected by e-prescribing. It would be ideal if somehow this information could be readily available for physicians and pharmacists, but it is highly unlikely that this will happen anytime soon, regardless of implementation of e-prescribing.

Although pharmacists are seen as the gatekeepers for patients to obtain prescription drugs, patients can obtain prescription medications from other pharmacies and/or from dispensing physicians. Patients also may borrow from friends, relatives, or even casual acquaintances. In addition, patients obtain OTC medications from physicians through prescriptions, on advice from pharmacists, through self-selection, or through the recommendations of friends or acquaintances. Through all of this, it must be recognized that both formal (structural) and informal (pervasive) system components are at play. Pharmacists or physicians may or may not be consulted regarding the use of medications. But, in some cases, health professionals are unaware of the drugs patients are taking. In addition, herbal remedies or health supplements may be taken without the knowledge or input of a health professional.

As an example, consider the patient medication profiling capability of most pharmacists. Computerization of patient medication records is commonplace in pharmacies. This computerization allows for the following:

- Ease in billing third-party prescription programs
- Maintenance of drug allergy information
- Drug use review
- Notification of drug interactions
- Aid in meeting the OBRA'90 (Omnibus Budget Reconciliation Act of 1990) requirements for patient counseling, drug use review, and estimation of appropriateness of therapy

This computerization permits drug-related information to be easily entered, retained, and retrieved. However, OTC medications are rarely entered into such records. (One exception may be OTC drugs prescribed by physicians and dispensed through a prescription by pharmacists.) This exclusion of a whole class of drugs from the monitoring programs of pharmacies may have a profound effect upon the ability of pharmacists to monitor the drug therapies of their patients. If the patient purchases the OTC medication in the pharmacy, the pharmacist may have an idea of the drugs consumed; however, if OTC drugs are purchased in a nonpharmacy outlet, the pharmacist is completely unaware of many drugs a patient may be taking. Another factor adding to the complexity of the problem is the fact that a patient may also utilize numerous pharmacies for varying prescription products. Thus there is no one record repository for all medications a patient may be taking. e-Prescribing will have little or no effect on this missing segment to access patient drug use that is self-medication in nature.

Noncompliance as a Patient Response to Prescriptions
Patients are noncompliant purposefully in many settings, including hospitals where administration of medications is routine.[2] In the ambulatory setting, noncompliance can be on purpose or incidental.[3] Patients may make such noncompliant decisions based upon many factors that may include their individual health beliefs, lack of faith in prescribers or therapy prescribed, occurrence of ADRs, or depression due to the realization of the need for a long-term therapy.

Hughes takes the view that patient noncompliance by seniors may in fact be "intelligent noncompliance" to avoid adverse effects or lack of therapeutic benefit.[4] In some cases, by self-monitoring of conditions or symptoms, patients may feel that it may not be necessary for them to continue to take medications. Some drugs are prescribed on an as-needed basis. Examples here might be oral antihistamines for allergies that may vary during the year and may not need to be taken year round. In another instance, the dose of a drug such as insulin to treat diabetes may require an alteration in the amount injected or a decision whether it is to be taken via an insulin pump.

Another factor leading to noncompliance with seniors, or other patients for that matter, is economically driven. The cost aspect of noncompliance should not be understated, and it certainly has an ethical component as well. Ethics relate to manufacturers' profit-driven ethos, driving patients to be noncompliant due to the high cost of pharmacotherapy.

Also, a patient may need to alter how they take a drug, such as digoxin to treat congestive heart failure if their pulse falls below a certain minimum amount. The dosing of many drugs is more art than science and may require that patients be intelligently noncompliant with prescribed therapies.

The Impact of Insurance Coverage or Lack Thereof
External variables may greatly influence patients and their drug taking behaviors. Coverage for prescribed drugs allows those with coverage to obtain medications

with varying cost-sharing requirements; however, many do not have insurance coverage for drugs or other health-related needs. It has been estimated that 15% of Americans, approximately 47 million people, lacked health insurance for all or part of the current year. Certainly, these considerations have huge ramifications on how and when consumers obtain prescribed and OTC medications. Even if consumers do happen to have insurance coverage for prescription drugs, the co-pays and deductibles may still be too expensive for consumers.

The gap in coverage for Medicare enrollees in the Medicare Part D drug benefit is another example of coverage not necessarily meeting all patients' needs. The so-called "donut hole" after initial coverage for prescription drugs, followed by a period where there is no coverage, and finally reaching catastrophic coverage forces many seniors to make extremely difficult decisions pertaining to the use of both prescription and OTC drugs.

Patient Safety

Medication errors are common, costly, and injurious to patients.[5] Often, pediatric patients suffer more significant adverse drug events than do adults.[5] e-Prescribing and health IT offers the hope that more precise dosing for small bodies can occur with the use of these technologies. Pediatric patients suffer perhaps more so because, as potent drugs are used with smaller volumes of distribution of drugs and with immature kidney and liver metabolism of drugs, the potential for dosing errors can increase.[5]

Evidence-based medicine (EBM) refers to the use of the current best accepted evidence when making decisions about care for patients. EBM guidelines enabled by health IT and provided through e-prescribing systems have been shown to increase patient safety and reduce morbidity associated with medication errors.[6]

e-Prescribing features such as automated reminders for physicians regarding patient specific information, duplication alerts, and other prescribed therapies have increased prescribing efficiency and effectiveness.[7] In a British study of the effects of e-prescribing on the quality of prescribing, findings pointed to an enhancement of the quality of prescribing and thus an increase in patient safety.[8]

The use of EMRs enhance safety due to the ease of access of patient information readily stored and readily available for prescriber use in current prescribing activities.[9] Kaelber and Bates point to the enhancement of patient safety enabled by the exchange of patient-specific health information to other health care providers.[10] Many aspects of health care delivery can be improved by EMRs, e-prescribing, and the exchange of electronically based health information, but the aspect of improving patient safety by electronically mediated methods holds the most promise for enabling a more focused delivery of services to patients.

e-Prescribing to the Rescue

With the advent of new, sophisticated IT, such as e-prescribing, pharmacists working with physicians and other prescribers should be able to harness computer technology so as to better monitor drug use and the drug use process regardless of patient access to medications. Within PBMs, state Medicaid programs, and CMS through Medicare, analysts can better examine population-based indices of a drug or a drug class's worth. Outcomes, both economic and therapeutic, can be tracked with much greater efficiency than is currently possible. How is this possible? With these varying systems meshing comes the possibility of an easier collapsing of data into one set as opposed to separate sets that at present are unable to be combined into a unitary database.

Patient Satisfaction with e-Prescribing

British Experiences

Researchers in the United Kingdom have examined physicians' (general practitioners'), pharmacists', and patients' satisfaction of electronic transfer of prescription related information, including e-prescribing.[11] Each of the three sampled groups expressed satisfaction with e-prescribing. Porteous et al noted that patients specifically felt that e-prescribing would provide an improvement in the convenience of obtaining prescriptions from pharmacies.[11] It is interesting to note that in this study, both the sample of general practitioners and patients were concerned about pharmacists having access to general medical records that did not specifically relate to prescriptions and medication-related issues.[11] This will be an important factor to consider and deal with both in the United Kingdom as well as the United States. This potential reluctance on the part of patients will require focused educational efforts to have patients understand the importance of access to medical records by pharmacists as well as others on the health care team. Medical records that are all encompassing have been shared by all health providers in institutional settings for decades with wide access to all professionals. It is always useful to have an appreciation of what issues are involved for all stakeholders when considering adoption of new technologies (i.e., e-prescribing).

United States Experience with Patient Satisfaction

The U.S. Secretary of HHS points to enhancement of patient satisfaction with e-prescribing.[12] Leavitt notes:[12(p.28)]

> Patient satisfaction is another important component driving e-prescribing. Even if e-prescribing improves prescriber workflow, if patients report problems when they go to pick up a prescription, prescriber adoption may be limited. Only one site, SureScripts, included this outcome in their study. They found that of the 834 patients surveyed, 56 percent either moderately or strongly preferred e-prescribing over paper prescriptions. Adults under 65 years of age were 2.2 times more likely to strongly prefer e-prescribing. However, due to the limited experience of the pilot sites in this area, further study is warranted.

Enhanced Communication

In a descriptor of how e-medicine has improved his patients' satisfaction, Stone notes that a system set up in his practice allowed for online appointment scheduling, electronic prescription refills, general messaging capabilities, and "Web visits" with physicians.[13] Appropriate caution necessitated ensuring a definite secure Web access and messaging system; to not do this would violate Health Insurance Portability and Accountability Act (HIPAA) guidelines. Stone also points out that some insurers—Aetna, Cigna, and others—now reimburse physicians for Web visits in Florida, California, Massachusetts, and New York.[13]

Ease of Access, Contact with Physicians

Patients who use these systems are delighted with ease of access and the ability to contact physicians directly, to receive information in a timely fashion, and/or to avoid the distressing challenges of a telephone tree/triage setup requiring patience and time.

Enhanced Communication Leading to Enhanced Care

Kilbridge points to numerous benefits for patients in e-prescribing.[14] They include enhanced safety of medication management process and perhaps an increase in compliance due to a "closed loop" communication process between payers and providers (physicians and pharmacists). Also noted is a potential for improved efficiencies. Automated formulary checking can enable better adherence to formulary guidelines and can avoid delays, which are common in paper, facsimile, and other antiquated systems currently in use.[14]

Patients Pushing Their Physicians into the Brave New World of e-Communicating in Health Care

In fact, in 2000 Kassirer suggested: "Many patients are beginning to use online communications and are dragging their doctors along."[15(p.116)] Patients obtain much information from Web-based sources at present, so it is reasonable to assume that information from their own caregivers will be in demand as soon as they can access physicians in this manner. Many technology companies working with insurers, employers, providers, and patients enable patients to access pertinent information in a secure portal. This information may relate to drugs, diseases, or preventive type health activities. The dynamic in place between patients and physicians in an e-mediated world will be different than that in place at present. Patience is always a virtue when implementing any new technology for patients; e-prescribing will undoubtedly require patience by all, and most importantly by patients.

Summary

e-Prescribing will produce immediate effects for patients. Some of these will be noticed; many may not be apparent. Regardless of initial recognition or not, patients will soon benefit and realize the benefits of a streamlined, efficient, and safer process for obtaining prescriptions than that currently available.

Seamless Process

In many ways, a move to an e-prescribing platform should be a seamless process for patients. They need to seek care by contacting physicians, but therapeutic plans should unfold for patients in a manner that does not alter dramatically how care plans are followed through upon. In fact, patients may be unaware of how the system differs from current systems.

Convenience Will Be Palpable

The system's enabling of a more convenient approach to receiving prescriptions will not escape the eye of patients. This should be real and affect individuals immediately.

Decrease in Adverse Drug Events

A decrease in potential ADEs could ensue. Patients do not necessarily expect ADEs at present, so their absence will be welcome certainly but not necessarily perceived as being attributable to e-prescribing systems.

Initial Compliance

Initial rates of noncompliance are estimated to be upwards of 20% at present in the United States. This means that one-fifth of all new prescriptions are never filled by patients after going through the process of seeking care, seeing a physician, receiving a prescription order, and having the order in place for processing by pharmacists. e-Prescribing technologies will identify initial noncompliers and can have notices sent to the prescriber, the pharmacy, and the patient.

Enhanced Choices for Patients

Additional benefits for patients include the ability to get the most out of their pharmacy. By indicating generic availability and formulary inclusion, physicians can more accurately help patients obtain the best value for their prescription expenditures. Patients can save time by indicating to the physician which pharmacy to use for their prescription transmittals. This alone will save time because the patient will undoubtedly know immediately which pharmacy will have the prescription.

Benefits Should Be Apparent

It is hard to not see the benefits for patients with e-prescribing. The very real benefits of decreased medication errors; enhanced prescription record keeping and access; and the great benefit of increased convenience will be universally hailed by patients and patient advocates. Education of patients on what e-prescribing is and what it is not will be crucial for acceptance and eventual satisfaction. Patience is always a virtue when implementing any new technology for patients. e-Prescribing will undoubtedly require patience by all, most importantly patients.

References

1. Fincham J. Pharmacists, patients, and professional roles. *Harvard Health Pol Rev.* 2006; 7(1):169–179.
2. Canada AT, Lesko LJ. Two reasons for unusual therapeutic drug monitoring results in hospitalized patients. *Ther Drug Monit.* 1980;2(3):217–219.
3. Johnson MJ, Williams M, Marshal FS. Adherent and nonadherent medication-taking in elderly hypertensive patients. *Clin Nurs Res.* 1999;8(4):318–335.
4. Hughes CM. Medication non-adherence in the elderly: how big is the problem? *Drugs Aging.* 2004;21(12):793–811.
5. Rainu Kaushal R, Barker KN, Bates DW. How can information technology improve patient safety and reduce medication errors in children's health care? *Arch Pediatr Adolesc Med.* 2001;155(9):1002–1007.
6. Leape LL, Berwick DM, Bates DW. What practices will most improve safety? Evidence-based medicine meets patient safety. *JAMA.* 2002;288(4):501–507.
7. Martens JD, van der Weijden T, Winkens RAG, et al. Feasibility and acceptability of a computerised system with automated reminders for prescribing behaviour in primary care. *Int J Med Inform.* 2008;77(3):199–207.
8. Donyai P, O'Grady K, Jacklin A, Barber, N, Franklin, BD. The effects of electronic pre-scribing on the quality of prescribing. *Br J Clin Pharmacol.* 2008;65(2):230–237.
9. Warren J. *General Practice EMRs: What They Can Tell Us and How.* December 2007. Available at: http://hcro.enigma.co.nz/website/index.cfm?fuseaction=articledisplay& FeatureID=011207. Accessed June 14, 2008.
10. Kaelber DC, Bates DW. Health information exchange and patient safety. *J Biomed Inform.* 2007;40(suppl 6):s40–s45.
11. Porteous T, Bond C, Robertson R, Hannaford P, Reiter E. Electronic transfer of prescrip-tion-related information: comparing views of patients, general practitioners, and pharma-cists. *Br J Gen Pract.* 2003;53(488):204–209.
12. Leavitt MO. *Pilot testing of initial electronic prescribing standards—cooperative agree-ments required under section 1860D-(4)(e) of the Social Security Act as amended by the Medicare Prescription Drug, Improvement, and Modernization Action (MMA) of 2003.* Available at: http://www.cms.hhs.gov/EPrescribing. Accessed November 24, 2007.
13. Stone JH. Communication between physicians and patients in the era of e-medicine. *N Engl J Med.* 2007;356(24):2451–2453.
14. Kilbridge P. *e-Prescribing.* Oakland, CA: California HealthCare Foundation; 2001.
15. Kassirer JP. Patients, physicians, and the Internet. *Health Aff.* 2000;19(6):115–123.

ELEVEN

What Do Physicians Need to Do Now?

Introduction

This chapter will outline the steps you need to take to ensure that your practice is ready to begin e-prescribing. The steps are simple and straightforward. None of these items should cause problems for you or your patients. Computer-to-computer transmission of prescriptions will become more commonplace in the near and long-term future.

Items to Consider

SureScripts has provided a guide for physicians to use when proceeding to implement e-prescribing options for their practice.[1] In *Your Guide to Electronic Prescribing*, it is suggested that these steps be followed:[1]

1. *Determine if your practice already uses technology that has been certified to connect with pharmacies.*

SureScripts suggests you may already be set up to begin e-prescribing.[1] It is estimated that at present 150,000 physicians are using e-prescribing or EMRs. The pharmacies listed in **Table 11-1** are set up to receive e-prescribing prescriptions.

TABLE 11-1   **Certified Pharmacies Enabled to Receive e-Prescribing Prescriptions**

Pharmacy

Acme	Longs Drug
Albertsons	Medicap pharmacies (independent community
Brooks	pharmacies)
CVS/pharmacy	The Medicine Shoppe Pharmacy
Duane Reade	Meijer Pharmacy
Eckerd	Osco Pharmacy
Familymeds Pharmacy	Pathmark
FredMeyer	Publix
Frys	Quality Food Centers
Giant	Ralphs
Giant Eagle Pharmacy	RiteAid
Good Neighbor Pharmacy (independent	Safeway
community pharmacies)	Sam's Club
Hannaford	SavMore
Happy Harrys	ShopRite
Harris Teater	Smith's
H-E-B Pharmacy	Stop & Shop
HyVee	Sweetbay
Jewel-Osco	Target
Local independent pharmacies	Times Pharmacy
Kash n' Karry	Ukrop's
Kerr Drug	Walgreens
Kroeger	Wal-Mart

These pharmacies are chain community, food market, and/or large (big box—Wal-Mart, Target, Sam's Club, etc.) pharmacies. Independent community pharmacies are not listed in this table. You will need to individually contact each independent community pharmacy to determine if they are set up to accept receipt of e-prescribing prescriptions. Also, some EMR systems have a module in place facilitating e-prescribing. You may already have a system in place that is ready to use.

   2. *Find out if your practice uses what is called a "certified solution."*

SureScripts suggests contacting the vendor providing your office technology solutions.[1] Let them know that you wish to enable e-prescribing—not just the ability to fax prescriptions to pharmacies. There may or may not be a system upgrade that is required for you to initiate e-prescribing. Ask if any training is provided or required, as well as determine if any of this will require extra fees on your part.

    3. *Acquire the e-prescribing technology for your practice.*

Find out if you are eligible for programs that are designed to entice physicians to set up e-prescribing in their practices. Examples of such programs include the following:

- Some state health departments
- Some payer group (e.g., Blue Cross–Blue Shield plans [Massachusetts, Michigan, and elsewhere])
- State medical associations
- Federal government (e.g., CMS)

Specific questions to ask include the following:

- Is there a cost for me to participate?
- Do I need to purchase anything?
- Are there fees, monthly maintenance, initial start-up costs, etc.?
- Is there training necessary, and is it extensive?
  - ○ What options for training are available for staff in my office?
- Can I deal with both new and refill prescriptions?
- Can the systems I have in my practice at present (such as demographics and lab values) mesh with the systems for e-prescribing?
- What types of services are most important to have in place?
  - ○ Electronic refills (e-refills: the ability to monitor and allow prescription refills via e-prescribing systems)
    - If you have refill e-prescribing capabilities, try and process these refill requests promptly. Avoid batch processing and transmittal at later times during the day.
    - Let your patients know that contacting their pharmacist continues to be the first step in obtaining refill prescriptions

○ Obtaining a history of current and past prescriptions from community/chain/institutional pharmacies

■ How willing is the computer vendor supplying the e-prescribing technology to deal with potential problems?

○ Can they provide references for assessing how well they provide support services?

○ What is the turnaround time for responding to problems?

○ What are your fall back mechanisms in case of failure of the e-prescribing system?

4. *Make sure that your current patient information that may be electronically stored can be pre-loaded into e-prescribing software options.*

5. *Find out which pharmacies in your practice catchment area are enabled for e-prescribing and notify them that you are ready to e-prescribe.*

Be sure that your patients are aware of this capability!

6. *Ensure that you are able to send your prescriptions electronically immediately.*

7. *Some prescriptions cannot be transmitted electronically at this time.*

■ DEA guidelines do not allow for electronic transmission of Schedule II prescriptions.

■ DEA regulations do not allow electronic signatures for Schedule III–V drugs at this time. These prescriptions will need your hand signature and then they can be transmitted via facsimile to pharmacies for processing. The facsimile transmissions cannot be computer generated with your electronic signature. You will need to sign these prescriptions by hand and then send.

8. *Glitches may invariably occur.*

I suggest dry runs to test all the capabilities. Above all else, make sure the supplying vendor for the e-prescribing technology is kept abreast of any and all problems immediately when they occur. It goes without saying that all on your staff need to be aware of how to contact the supplying vendor!

What Does Reality Tell Us About Physicians and Commercial e-Prescribing Systems?

Although great progress is currently seen in physician experiences with commercial e-prescribing systems, there are problematic areas that need to be addressed continually.[2] Grossman et al have reported on a study of 44 participating physicians between November 2005 and March 2006.[3]

Identified Items Needing Improvement

Availability of Systems

It has been estimated by Blumenthal and colleagues that in 2006, a total of 4% to 24% of hospitals presently have CPOE, which the authors state is the best proxy for inpatient EHR adoption.[4]

Variation in e-Prescribing Systems

In the Grossman et al study, two-thirds of the practices used a module for e-prescribing contained in an EMR system.[3] A total of one-third used a stand-alone e-prescribing system.[5]

Complete Patient Medication Listings

Maintenance of a complete patient medication database was noted in the Grossman et al study as an obstacle hindering e-prescribing.[3] As was noted earlier in this book, the lack of a complete profile for medications for patients occurs with any system—paper based, electronic profiles in pharmacies, and EHRs. This needs to be remedied before e-prescribing can reach its full potential. In some cases, patient records of prescriptions were manually loaded into EHR systems; this is costly both in terms of time and resources. Discontinued medications or medications that are used by patients that fall outside of formulary requirements but are still prescribed may not show up on EHRs.

Clinical Decision Support

Physicians reported that the clinical support features were not optimally complete in some EHR systems.[5] For example, only 20% of reporting physicians indicated their EHR system did not have complete drug-condition interaction capabilities. Half of the reporting physicians indicated that they had drug-allergy contraindication capability.

Patient Specific Formulary Information

One of the key selling points of e-prescribing is the ability to refer to formulary requirements for patients online. In the Grossman et al study, slightly less than 50% of the practices had adequate patient health plan formulary information readily available.[4]

Cost of Implementation

Conn writes that in a survey of 5,000 physicians, 66% of the physicians without EHR indicated lack of financing was an obstacle to implementing EHRs, and 36% of those with a functioning EHR system indicated some financing of systems would be helpful.[5] Wilder suggests that to initially set up an EHR system $44,000 is required per physician with an additional $8,500 annual maintenance fee.[6]

EHRs Hinder Productivity

A surprising 27% of responders in the Conn study with EHR systems pointed to a lack of productivity that occurred with EHRs.[5]

Clinical Data Exchange Across Differing Provider Organizations

Regional Health Information Organizations (RHIOs) are organizations that support the electronic interchange of health information from one independent entity to another. The structure of RHIOs varies from one part of the United States to another. Some RHIOs are privately owned, and others are government-sponsored. There were approximately 145 RHIOs identified in early 2007 by Adler-Milstein et al.[7] In a study of the current state of RHIOs, researchers found the following:[6]

- Twenty-five percent of the identified RHIOs were defunct in early 2007.
- Twenty of the 145 RHIOs could be considered to be of modest size.
- Grant and/or governmental funding is a necessity for RHIO continuation, in effect leading to a market-based approach to RHIO development.
- Type of data exchanged included the following:
  - Test results
    - Laboratory
    - Radiology
  - Medication histories
  - Outpatient data
  - Public health reports

Positive Features Experienced by Current Physician e-Prescribers

Prescribing Safety and Quality

To a person, respondents in the Grossman et al study indicated that prescribing safety and enhanced quality while enhancing their practice efficiency were crucial positive features associated with e-prescribing.[4]

Practice Efficiency

As just noted, enhancement of practice efficiency is one of the hallmarks of e-prescribing.[4] Avoiding legibility problems is a tangible and beneficial outcome of e-prescribing. Callbacks from pharmacies to physicians can drain productivity quickly; e-prescribing effectively eliminates the need for callbacks.

Summary

Effective guides to steer physicians easily into e-prescribing are available. These helpful summaries can provide information necessary to move forward with e-prescribing. About one-fourth of physicians are estimated to be using EHRs.[8] As more and more e-prescribing uses are documented and the volume of e-prescribed prescriptions continue to increase, the full benefit of e-prescribing as a means of electronically transforming the practice of medicine will no doubt continue to unfold.

It Can Be Done!

During the aftermath of the terrible devastation of Hurricane Katrina, a glimmer of joy could be realized by the fact that in an unprecedented fashion, health providers (physicians, pharmacies, health systems, governmental entities [Medicare and Medicaid]) provided seamless care using health IT to a degree previously thought impossible. If such success can be reached in the midst of such a disaster, similar implementation successes can be achieved elsewhere on a broad scale!

References

1. SureScripts. *Your Guide to Electronic Prescribing.* Available at: http://www.surescripts.com/pdf/Guide%20to%20EPrescribing%201.14.08lr.pdf. Accessed January 28, 2008.

2. Lapane K. Progress in e-prescribing [e-letters]. *Health Aff.* April 18, 2007;Web exclusive. Available at: http://content.healthaffairs.org/cgi/eletters/26/3/w393. Accessed June 19, 2008.

3. Grossman JM, Gerland A, Reed MC, Fahlman C. Physicians' experiences using commercial e-prescribing systems. *Health Aff.* April 3, 2007;26(3):w393–w404. Available at: doi: 10.1377/hlthaff.26.3.w393.

4. Blumenthal D, DesRoches C, Donelan K, et al. *Health Information Technology in the United States: The Information Base for Progress.* New York: The Robert Wood Johnson Foundation; 2006.

5. Conn J. Survey: financial support is no. 1 for EHR adoption. *Mod Healthcare.* Available at: http://www.modernhealthcare.com/apps/pbcs.dll/article?AID=/20080124/REG/435331572/1029/FREE. Accessed January 24, 2008.

6. Wilder BL. Adoption of open-sourced EHR technology leads to efficiencies, safety and quality care. *Advance for Health Information Executives.* 2007;11(8):49–54.

7. Adler-Milstein J, McAfee AP, Bates DW, Jha AK. The state of regional health information organizations: current activities and financing. *Health Aff.* 2007;Web exclusive:w60–w69.

8. Jha AK, Ferris TG, Konelan K, et al. How common are electronic health records in the United States? a summary of the evidence. *Health Aff.* 2006;Web exclusive:w496–w507.

APPENDIX A

Federal Law Mandating e-Prescribing

Electronic Prescription Drug Program

- The Secretary shall promulgate final standards for electronic prescribing no later than April 1, 2008. The final standards will follow a set of initial standards (to be issued no later than September 1, 2005) and a 1-year pilot project for the initial standards that begins January 1, 2006. The National Committee on Vital and Health Statistics—expanded to include representatives of physicians, pharmacists, and experts on e-prescribing, among others—will consult with standard-setting organizations and may recommend standards to the Secretary.

- Within 1 year of the promulgation of the final standards, any prescriptions for covered part D drugs prescribed for Medicare beneficiaries that are transmitted electronically must be transmitted according to those standards.

Source: Centers for Medicare and Medicaid Studies. *Summary of H.R. 1: Medicare Prescription Drug, Improvement, and Modernization Act of 2003* (Public Law 108-173). April 2004. Available at: http://www.cms.hhs.gov/MMAUpdate/downloads/PL108-173 summary.pdf. Accessed May 27, 2008.

- The new e-prescribing standards should be designed to enable transmission of basic prescription data to and from doctors and pharmacists, as well as information about the patient's drug utilization history, possible drug interactions, the drug plan (including information about the formulary and cost-sharing), and information about lower-cost therapeutically appropriate alternatives. The standards must comply with HIPAA privacy rules. Messaging unrelated to appropriate prescribing (such as marketing) will not be allowed.

- The Secretary, in consultation with the Attorney General, will develop safe harbors under the anti-kickback and physician self-referral laws, allowing hospitals, group practices, PDPs, and MA plans to provide physicians with nonmonetary remuneration, in the form of hardware, software, information technology services and training, which is necessary and used solely for electronic prescribing.

APPENDIX B

A Recent Timeline for the Implementation of e-Prescribing

Over the last four years, several private organizations, states, and regional collaboratives have sought to implement and evaluate the effectiveness of integrated e-prescribing systems:

- In 2002, Tufts Health Plan of Massachusetts and Advance PCS (now Caremark) conducted a year-long pilot study of integrated e-prescribing. The study involved over 100 clinicians, and found that e-prescribing had positive effects on patient safety, cost, pharmacy and prescriber efficiency, and user satisfaction.
- In 2003, Blue Cross–Blue Shield of Massachusetts, in conjunction with various industry partners, launched the eRx Collaborative. The Collaborative's goal was to deploy e-prescribing systems in the offices of 3,400 Massachusetts physicians. After two years, the program had allowed for

Adapted from: The National Opinion Research Center (NORC) at the University of Chicago. *Findings from the Evaluation of e-Prescribing Pilot Sites* (AHRQ Publication No. 07-0047-EF). Chicago: April 2007. This document is in the public domain.

over three million prescriptions to be transmitted electronically. With regards to safety, by 2005 more than 5,500 prescriptions per month were being changed as a result of warning messages built into the system.

- In 2003, the Rhode Island Quality Institute started a program to implement statewide e-prescribing throughout the state of Rhode Island. Aided by the state's appropriation of $20 million towards Health Information Exchange, as well as underwriting from e-prescribing network SureScripts and vendor LighthouseMD, the public, private, and academic partnership was met with great success. In 2006, Rhode Island was ranked first in the country in e-prescribing.

- In 2003, the Massachusetts Medical Society developed a strategic plan for implementing interoperable e-prescribing throughout the state of Massachusetts. Later, in 2005, the society subsidized e-prescribing for its members. Massachusetts was recently ranked third in e-prescribing, according to pharmacy groups.

- In 2004, Wellpoint, Inc. of Indiana introduced the Physician Quality and Technology Initiative (PQTI). The program gave e-prescribing and administrative software to over 19,000 physicians in HMOs and PPOs in California, Georgia, Missouri, and Wisconsin. Although the majority of physicians enrolled in this program use only the administrative software program, the preliminary results surrounding e-prescribing are encouraging. As of July 2005, over 90,000 prescriptions had been written electronically, and offices using the e-prescribing utility were spending 75% less time on administrative work.

- In 2004, CareFirst Blue Cross Blue Shield, Maryland's largest insurer, decided to provide DrFirst's Rcopia to 500 physicians. CareFirst and DrFirst also gave wireless handheld devices developed by spring and palmOne Inc. to participating physicians. After the program's first year, it was estimated that over $1.3 million in cost savings could be directly attributed to reduced prescribing errors.

- In 2005, Blue Cross–Blue Shield of Michigan and the big three American automakers joined forces with local pharmacy benefit managers and HMOs to launch the Southeast Michigan e-Prescribing Initiative (SEMI). Over 17,000 physicians had the opportunity to participate in the program, which successfully developed an interoperable e-prescribing system throughout the region. Between August 2005 and April 2006, Henry Ford Medical Group reported over 588,000 electronic scripts in total, with 70,000 prescriptions canceled due to drug-drug interaction warnings and over 4,500 prescriptions canceled due to allergy alerts. In addition, over the course of the entire project, researchers found a net reduction in pharmacist initiated calls, as well as a savings in physician telephone time. Together, these efficiencies could save an estimate $2.9 billion per year. Other findings included increased formulary compliance rates and increased generic dispensing for physicians who used e-prescribing.

- In 2005, the state of Delaware launched a pilot e-prescribing program with 100 physicians, using the system Rcopia, developed by DrFirst. Results from the pilot study will be published in late 2006. As of June 2006, more than 75,426 prescriptions had been written electronically.

- In 2005, Sierra Health Services, it subsidiaries Health Plan of Nevada and Southwest Medical Associates (SMA), and the Clark County Medical Society of Nevada funded a program to provide all 5,000 physicians in the state with e-prescribing software. All Nevada physicians were eligible to receive a free license for Allscripts' Touchworks Rx+ application. Since the implementation of the application, use of generic drugs among patients increased from 59% of prescriptions written to 65%; this increase translates into an annual cost savings of $5 million. In addition, callbacks from pharmacies declined and patient satisfaction increased.

- In January 2006, Blue Cross–Blue Shield of North Carolina started "ePrescribe," an initiative that provided funding for e-prescribing software, hardware, and support for 1,000 physicians in North Carolina.

- In May 2006, L.A. Care, the largest Medicaid HMO in the country, began an e-prescribing pilot program. The Los Angeles-based health care payer purchased hardware and software from Zix Corporation and provided it free of charge to participating physicians. The initial pilot study involved 50 physicians, but may ultimately include as many as 100. In October 2006, New Hampshire Governor John Lynch announced the goal of having all doctors in his state prescribing electronically by 2008. According to experts, New Hampshire has a good chance of achieving this goal, due in part to its small size, as well as the fact that in 2006, New Hampshire already possessed a fairly advanced health information system—nearly

75% of the state's primary care physicians used EHRs, and up to 80% of the state's pharmacies had e-prescribing capabilities.

- In January 2007, a coalition of technology companies and healthcare organizations calling themselves the National e-prescribing Patient Safety Initiative announced a program aimed at providing free e-prescribing to every physician in America. The coalition is led by Allscripts and Dell, and includes Aetna, Cisco Systems, Fujitsu Computers of America, Google, Microsoft, Sprint Nextel, SureScripts, Wellpoint, and Wolters Kluwer Health. Through web-based software available for free at http://www.natinoalerx.com, the coalition hopes to appeal to small practice physicians who otherwise would not wish to purchase an e-prescribing system.

- In January 2007, TennCare, Tennessee's Medicaid program, received a $674,200 HHS grant to launch an electronic prescription system linking rural doctors and pharmacies. The main goals of the program are to reduce pharmacy costs and increase patient safety by providing physicians in rural communities with computers to transmit prescriptions to local pharmacies.

- In February 2007, five of Florida's largest health plans announced a joint effort to encourage the State's physicians to use e-prescribing. The collaborative, named "e-Prescribe Florida" involves Blue Cross–Blue Shield of Florida, Av-Med, Cigna, Humana, and UnitedHealthcare.

- December 2007, President George W. Bush reiterates the stated goal of an electronic health record for every American by 2014.

- The budget allocated for the Office of the National Coordinator for Health Information Technology is $61.3 million for the current fiscal year—the same amount the office got for fiscal 2007. This amount is reduced from the amount requested by the President of $117.9 million. This amounts to a decrease of 48% over what was initially proposed by the President.

APPENDIX C

Descriptions of Federal Laws for Protecting Personal Health Information

There are several federal statutes that protect personal health information. HIPAA provides the most extensive and specific protection. However, other federal statutes, although not always focused specifically on health information, nonetheless have the effect of protecting personal health information in specific situations. This table presents an outline of selected federal laws that protect personal health information.

Source: U.S. Government Accountability Office. *Health Information Technology. Early Efforts Initiated, but Comprehensive Privacy Approach Needed for National Strategy* (GAO-07-238). Washington, DC: January 2007. Available at: http://www.gao.gov/htext/d07238.html. Accessed May 28, 2008.

TABLE C-1

Law	Impact
HIPAA (HIPAA administrative simplification provisions and regulations)	*Protected information:* Certain individually identifiable health information transmitted by or maintained in electronic or any other form or medium by a covered entity. *Protection provided:* Disclosure of health information prohibited except as permitted by the Privacy Rule. The Security Rule requires that the security, integrity, and confidentiality of health information must be ensured. *Applicability:* Covered entities, which are defined as health plans, health care clearinghouses, and health care providers who transmit health information electronically in connection with authorized transactions.

Privacy protections applicable to federal government agencies:

Law	Impact
Privacy Act of 1974	*Protected information:* Agency-controlled information about an individual that is retrieved using the individual's name or other personal identifier. *Protection provided:* Prohibits use and disclosure of personal records without consent of individual, or as otherwise permitted under the law; also requires protection of personal records, disclosure of which could cause harm, embarrassment, unfairness, or inconvenience to the individual. *Applicability:* Executive agencies that hold information in a system of records (the law provides certain exceptions).
Freedom of Information Act of 1966	*Protected information:* Federal agency records. *Protection provided:* Act exempts from public release individually identifiable medical information, disclosure of which would constitute a clearly unwarranted invasion of personal privacy. *Applicability:* Executive federal agencies.

TABLE C-1 *(Continued)*

Law	*Impact*
Social Security Act	*Protected information:* Individually identifiable records and information held by an agency regarding program beneficiaries' records and information that is transmitted to, or obtained by or from HHS, Social Security Administration (SSA), and their contractors incident to carrying out agency duties. *Protection provided:* Prohibits unauthorized disclosure of individually identifiable records and makes unauthorized disclosure a crime. *Applicability:* HHS, SSA, and their contractors.
Veterans Omnibus Health Care Act of 1976	*Protected information:* Confidential medical records of treatment relating to the treatment of drug abuse, alcoholism or alcohol abuse, infection with the human immunodeficiency virus, or sickle cell anemia. *Protection provided:* Personally identifiable patient information provided or obtained in connection with treatment, education, evaluation, or research of certain conditions or diseases must be kept confidential, except with patient's written consent, or within VA, Department of Justice, or DOD. *Applicability:* VA.

Provisions protecting health information in limited situations:

Medicare Prescription Drug, Improvement, and Modernization Act of 2003	*Protected information:* Program beneficiaries' prescription drug, medication, and medical history information. *Protection provided:* Prescription drug plan sponsors must comply with HIPAA Privacy Rule and Security Rule requirements. *Applicability:* Prescription drug plan pharmacies and sponsors of prescription drug plans.

(continues)

TABLE C-1 *(Continued)*

Law	*Impact*
Clinical Laboratory Improvement Amendments of 1988	*Protected information:* Medical information of patients and clinical study subjects. *Protection provided:* Certain clinical laboratories are required to ensure confidentiality of test results or reports and may disclose such information only to authorized persons as defined by state or federal law. *Applicability:* Certain clinical laboratories conducting patient tests.
Public Health Service Act Health Omnibus Programs Extension of 1988	*Protected information:* Personal identifying information of individual subjects of biomedical, behavioral, clinical, or other research. *Protection provided:* The Secretary of HHS may issue a certificate of confidentiality to researchers engaged in biomedical, behavioral, clinical, or other research to protect any identifying research information from disclosure, including "compulsory legal demands." *Applicability:* Research programs.
Public Health Service Act Federal Confidentiality Requirements for Substance Abuse Patient Records	*Protected information:* Patient alcohol and drug abuse treatment records. *Protected provided:* Personally identifiable patient records maintained in connection with performance of drug abuse or substance abuse treatment must be kept confidential, absent patient consent or court order. *Applicability:* Federally assisted alcohol or substance abuse programs or activities.
Family Educational Rights and Privacy Act; Protection of Pupil Rights Amendment (education records are excluded under HIPAA's privacy and security regulations)	*Protected information:* Personally identifiable information in students' educational records; examination, testing, or treatment for mental or psychological conditions. *Protection provided:* Prohibits disclosure of protected information other than as needed within educational institution or by local or

TABLE C-1   *(Continued)*

Law	*Impact*
	state educational agency, absent consent of parent, or student that has reached 18 years of age. *Applicability:* Educational institution or agency that receives federal funds under the Department of Education programs; educational institutions that conduct non-Department of Education-funded surveys.
Americans with Disabilities Act	*Protected information:* Medical information or condition and health records of employees or applicants. *Protection provided:* Covered entities must treat employees' and applicants' medical information as confidential medical records, with certain limitations as specified in the law. *Applicability:* Employers of 15 or more employees, employment agencies, labor organizations, and joint labor management committees.
Financial Modernization (Gramm-Leach-Bliley) Act of 1999	*Protected information:* Nonpublic personal information, which is defined as any nonpublic personal financial information provided by a consumer to a financial institution. *Protection provided:* Prohibits disclosure of consumers' nonpublic personal information to nonaffiliated third parties without clients' consent. (Consumers must be afforded the opportunity to decline the institution's sharing their information with nonaffiliated third parties.) *Applicability:* Financial institutions, including certain health insurers.

APPENDIX D

Medicare Program: Proposed Standards for e-Prescribing Under Medicare Part D*

I. Background

A. Legislative History

Section 101 of the Medicare Prescription Drug, Improvement, and Modernization Act of 2003 (MMA) (Pub.L. 108-173) amended title XVIII of the Social Security Act (the Act) to establish a voluntary prescription drug benefit program.

Prescription Drug Plan (PDP) sponsors and Medicare Advantage (MA) organizations offering Medicare Advantage-Prescription Drug Plans (MA-PD), are required to establish electronic prescription drug programs to provide for electronic transmittal of certain information to the prescribing provider and dispensing pharmacy and pharmacist. This would include information about eligibility, benefits (including drugs included in the applicable formulary, any tiered

---

*Only selected sections are listed here.

Source: U.S. Government Accountability Office. *Department of Health and Human Services, Centers for Medicare and Medicaid Services—Medicare Program: Standards for e-Prescribing Under Medicare Part D and Identification of Backward Compatible Version of Adopted Standard for E-Prescribing and the Medicare Prescription Drug Program* (Version 8.1) (GAO-08-690R). Washington, DC; April 23, 2008.

formulary structure and any requirements for prior authorization), the drug being prescribed or dispensed and other drugs listed in the medication history, as well as the availability of lower cost, therapeutically appropriate alternatives (if any) for the drug prescribed. The MMA directed the Secretary to promulgate uniform standards for the electronic transmission of such data.

There is no requirement that prescribers or dispensers implement e-prescribing. However, prescribers and dispensers who electronically transmit prescription and certain other information for covered drugs prescribed for Medicare Part D eligible beneficiaries, directly or through an intermediary, would be required to comply with any applicable final standards that are in effect.

Section 1860D-4(e)(4) of the Act generally required the Secretary to conduct a pilot project to test initial standards recognized under 1860D-4(e)(4)(A) of the Act, prior to issuing the final standards in accordance with section 1860D-4(e)(4)(D) of the Act. The initial standards were recognized by the Secretary in 2005 and then tested in a pilot project during calendar year (CY) 2006. The MMA created an exception to the requirement for pilot testing of standards where, after consultation with the National Committee on Vital and Health Statistics (NCVHS), the Secretary determined that there already was adequate industry experience with the standard(s). The first set of such standards, the "foundation standards," were recognized and adopted through notice and comment rulemaking as final standards without pilot testing. See 70 FR 67568.

Based upon the evaluation of the pilot project, and not later than April 1, 2008, the Secretary is required to issue final uniform standards under section 1860D-4(e)(4)(D). These final standards must be effective not later than 1 year after the date of their issuance.

In the e-prescribing final rule at 70 FR 67589, we also discussed the estimated start-up costs for e-prescribing for providers and/or dispensers. Based on industry input, we cited approximately $3,000 for annual support, maintenance, infrastructure and licensing costs.

Physicians at that time reported paying user-based licensing fees ranging from $80 to $400 per month. For further discussion of the start-up costs associated with e-prescribing, see the regulatory impact analysis section of this proposed regulation, and the e-prescribing final rule at 70 FR 67589.

For a further discussion of the statutory basis for this proposed rule and the statutory requirements at section 1860D-4(e) of the Act, please refer to section I.

(Background) of the E-Prescribing and the Prescription Drug Program proposed rule, published February 4, 2005 (70 FR 6256).

B. Regulatory History

In the e-prescribing final rule at 70 FR 67589, we also discussed the estimated start-up costs for e-prescribing for providers and/or dispensers. Based on industry input, we cited approximately $3,000 for annual support, maintenance, infrastructure and licensing costs. Physicians at that time reported paying user-based licensing fees ranging from $80 to $400 per month. For further discussion of the start-up costs associated with e-prescribing, see the regulatory impact analysis section of this proposed regulation, and the e-prescribing final rule at 70 FR 67589.

In the November 7, 2005 final rule, we addressed the issues of privacy and security relative to e-prescribing in general. We noted that disclosures of protected health information (PHI) in connection with e-prescribing transactions would have to meet the minimum necessary requirements of the Privacy Rule if the entity is a covered entity (70 FR 6161). It is important to note that health plans, prescribers, and dispensers are HIPAA covered entities, and that these covered entities under HIPAA must continue to abide by the applicable HIPAA standards including these for privacy and security. E-prescribing provisions do not affect or alter the applicability of the Privacy Act to a particular entity. Entities which are covered by the Privacy Act and the HIPAA Privacy Rule must comply with provisions of both. Entities are responsible for determining whether they fall under the Privacy Act.

We continue to agree that privacy and security are important issues related to e-prescribing. Achieving the benefits of e-prescribing require the prescriber and dispenser to have access to patient medical information that may not have been previously available to them.

Section 1860-D (e)(2) (C) of the Act requires that disclosure of patient data in e-prescribing must, at a minimum, comply with HIPAA's privacy and security requirements.

Although HIPAA standards for privacy and security are flexible and scalable to each entity's situation, they provide comprehensive protections. We will continue to evaluate additional standards for consideration as adopted e-prescribing standards. For further discussion of privacy and security and e-prescribing, refer to the final rule at 70 FR 67581 through 82.

1. Foundation Standards

After consulting with the NCVHS, the Secretary found that there was adequate industry experience with several potential e-prescribing standards. Upon adoption through notice and comment rulemaking, these standards were called "foundation" standards, because they would be the first set of final standards adopted for an electronic prescription drug program. Three standards were adopted for purposes of e-prescribing in the E-Prescribing and the Prescription Drug Program final rule, published November 7, 2005 (70 FR 67568). Two of these standards, Accredited Standards Committee (ASC) X12N 270/271; and The National Council for Prescription Drug Programs (NCPDP) Telecommunication Standard Specification, Version 5, Release 1 (Version 5.1), were previously adopted under the Health Insurance Portability and Accountability Act of 1996 (HIPAA) and have been in effect since 2001.

These foundation standards are as follows:

For the exchange of eligibility information between prescribers and Medicare Part D sponsors: Accredited Standards Committee (ASC) X12N 270/271—Health Care Eligibility Benefit Inquiry and Response, Version 4010, May 2000, Washington Publishing Company, 004010X092 and Addenda to Health Care Eligibility Benefit Inquiry and Response, Version 4010A1, October 2002, Washington Publishing Company. 004010X092A1 (hereafter referred to as the ASC X12N 270/271 standard).

For the exchange of eligibility inquiries and responses between dispensers and Medicare Part D sponsors: The National Council for Prescription Drug Programs (NCPDP) Telecommunication Standard Specification, Version 5, Release 1 (Version 5.1), September 1999, and equivalent NCPDP Batch Standard Batch Implementation Guide, Version 1,

Release 1 (Version 1.1), January 2000 supporting Telecommunications Standard Implementation Guide Version 5, Release 1 (Version 5.1) for NCPDP Data Record in the Detail Data Record (hereafter referred to as the NCPDP Telecommunications Standard).

For the exchange of new prescriptions, changes, renewals, cancellations and certain other transactions between prescribers and dispensers: NCPDP SCRIPT Standard, Implementation Guide, Version 5, Release 0 (Version 5.0), May 12, 2004, excluding the Prescription Fill Status Notification Transaction (and its three business cases; Prescription Fill Status Notification Transaction—Filled, Prescription Fill Status Notification Transaction—Not Filled, and Prescription Fill Status Notification Transaction—Partial Fill), hereafter referred to as NCPDP SCRIPT 5.0.

II. Provisions of the Proposed Rule

A. Proposed Retirement of NCPDP SCRIPT 5.0 and Adoption of NCPDP SCRIPT 8.1 as a Final Standard

We propose to revise §423.160(b)(1) to replace the NCPDP SCRIPT 5.0 standard with the NCPDP SCRIPT 8.1. Those providers and dispensers using e-prescribing to provide for the electronic communication of a prescription or prescription-related information would be required to use the NCPDP SCRIPT 8.1 for the following transactions:

- Get message transaction.
- Status response transaction.
- Error response transaction.
- New prescription transaction.
- Prescription change request transaction.
- Prescription change response transaction.
- Refill prescription request transaction.
- Refill prescription response transaction.
- Verification transaction.
- Password change transaction.
- Cancel prescription request transaction.
- Cancel prescription response transaction.

B. Proposed Adoption of an E-prescribing Standard for Medication History Transaction

In the Foundation Standards final rule, 70 FR 67568, we discussed the need for medication history standards, and that we were unaware of any standard for these transactions that clearly met the criteria for adequate industry experience. As a result, a standard for medication history was tested in the 2006 pilot project. The NCVHS noted in its September 2, 2004 letter to the Secretary that medication history information was communicated between payers and prescribers using proprietary messaging standards, frequently the Information File Transfer protocols established by RxHub, a national formulary and benefits information exchange.

The NCVHS recommended that HHS actively participate in and support the rapid development of an NCPDP standard for formulary and medication history using the RxHub protocol as a basis. In September 2005, RxHub announced that its propriety data transaction format for Medication History, which they had submitted to NCPDP, had been approved and incorporated into the NCPDP Script Standard, and approved by the American National Standard Institute (ANSI). NCVHS considered ANSI accreditation to be one criterion in their recommendation process for adoption of e-prescribing standards, and HHS adopted this as a criterion for determining adequate industry experience. (See 70 FR 67568, 67577 for a discussion of all the criterion considered by NCVHS.) The resulting NCPDP SCRIPT standard was recognized by the Secretary as an initial standard, then pilot tested in accordance with the MMA.

C. Proposed Adoption of an E-prescribing Standard for Formulary and Benefit Transactions

As a result of pilot testing, we are proposing to add §423.160(b)(4) to adopt the NCPDP Formulary and Benefit Standard 1.0, for the transaction of communicating formulary and benefit information between the prescriber and the plan sponsor when e-prescribing for covered Medicare Part D drugs for Medicare Part D eligible individuals. This standard is based on a proprietary file transfer protocol developed by RxHub, which is currently being used to communicate this information in many e-prescribing products. The RxHub protocols were submitted to NCPDP for accreditation, and the resulting standard was recognized by the Secretary as an initial standard and pilot-tested in accordance with the MMA.

The NCPDP Formulary and Benefits Standard 1.0 was implemented live in all pilot sites. This standard works in tandem with the eligibility request and response (ASC X12N 270/271). Once the individual is identified, the appropriate drug benefit coverage is located and transmitted to the requestor.

Adoption of this standard for formulary and benefits transactions between plan sponsors and prescribers may deliver added value in approximating patients' drug coverage and lead to patient-specific, real-time benefit information. The NCPDP Formulary and Benefits Standard 1.0 enables the prescriber to consider this information during the prescribing process, and make the most appropriate drug choice without extensive back-and-forth administrative activities with the pharmacy or the plan sponsors. As prescribers prescribe based on the coverage offered by a patient's plan formulary, plans will experience reduced costs through paying for drugs that are specific to their formularies for which they have negotiated favorable rates. Patients will see reduced costs in not having to pay increased out-of-pocket expenses for prescribed drugs that are not on their plan's formularies.

E. Proposed Compliance Date

In accordance with section 1860D-4(e) of the Act, the Secretary must issue certain final uniform standards for e-prescribing no later than April 1, 2008, to become effective not later than 1 year after the date of their promulgation. Therefore, in accordance with this requirement, the Secretary proposes a compliance date of 1 year after the publication of the final uniform standards. The Secretary also proposes adopting NCPDP SCRIPT 8.1 as the e-prescribing standard for the transactions listed in section III. C. of this proposed rule, effective 1 year after the publication of the final uniform standards. We solicit comments regarding the impact of these proposed dates on industry and other interested stakeholders and whether an earlier compliance date should be adopted.

III. Standards for an Electronic Prescribing Program (§423.160)

The emerging and increasing use of health care electronic data interchange (EDI) standards and transactions have raised the issue of the applicability of the PRA. It has been determined that a regulatory requirement mandating the use of a particular EDI standard constitutes an agency-sponsored third-party disclosure as defined under the PRA.

As a third-party disclosure requirement subject to the PRA, Medicare Part D sponsors offering qualified prescription drug coverage must support and comply with electronic prescription standards relating to covered Medicare Part D drugs, for Medicare Part D enrolled individuals as would be required under §423.160.

However, the requirement that Medicare Part D sponsors support electronic prescription drug programs in accordance with standards set forth in this section, as established by the Secretary, does not require that prescriptions be written or transmitted electronically by prescribers or dispensers. After the promulgation of this set of final standards, these entities will be required to comply with the proposed standards only if they transmit prescription information electronically as discussed in section 1860D-4(e)(1) and (2) of the Act.

Testimony presented to the NCVHS indicates that most health plans/PBMs currently have e-prescribing capability either directly or by contracting with another entity. Therefore, we do not believe that conducting an electronic prescription drug program would be an additional burden for those plans. We solicit industry and other interested stakeholder comments and input on this issue. Since these standards are already familiar to industry, we believe the requirement to adopt them constitutes a usual and customary business practice and the burden associated with the requirements is exempt from the PRA as stipulated under 5 CFR 1320.3(b)(2).

A. Overall Impact

According to 2006 CMS data, approximately 24 million beneficiaries were enrolled in a Medicare Part D plan enrolled in a Medicare Part D plan, (either a stand-alone Prescription Drug Plan or a Medicare Advantage Drug Plan). Another 7 million retirees were enrolled in employer or union-sponsored retiree drug coverage receiving the Retiree Drug Subsidy (RDS); 3 million in Federal retiree programs such as TRICARE and the Federal Employees Health Benefits Plans (FEHBP) and 5 million receiving drug coverage from alternative sources, including 2 million who have coverage through the Veterans' Administration. The breadth of Medicare's coverage suggests that e-prescribing under Medicare Part D could impact virtually every pharmacy and a large percentage of the physician practices in the country. Standards established for Medicare Part D beneficiaries will, as a matter of economic necessity, be adopted by vendors of e-prescribing and pharmacy software, and as a result, would extend to other populations unless they are manifestly unsuited for the purpose. However, we note again that e-prescribing is voluntary for both prescribers and dispensers under the Medicare Part D electronic prescribing program.

B. Costs

Because e-prescribing is voluntary, we anticipate that entities who currently do not now e-prescribe and who will not implement e-prescribing during the period reflected in the regulatory impact analysis will incur neither costs nor benefits.

Entities that do not now e-prescribe, but that will implement e-prescribing during the period reflected in the regulatory impact analysis will incur the costs and benefits associated with the foundation standards (which we discussed in the final rule at 70 FR 67568), but we do not claim either in this analysis. We assume that implementation of the NCPDP SCRIPT standards would not significantly affect the implementation cost; that is, the cost to implement the foundation standards and these two standards is not significantly higher than the cost of implementing the foundation standards alone. However, these entities could incur some additional costs for the purchase of new e-prescribing products that include these two transactions in the standard format. They would also incur the benefits of the two proposed standards. We solicit industry and other interested stakeholder comment and input on these issues.

We assume that since these standards are new and not currently deployed and implemented in vendor products, that entities do not exist that e-prescribe now and who have software that conducts these two transactions using the NCPDP SCRIPT standards.

Entities that e-prescribe now using a software product that cannot conduct the two transactions and cannot be upgraded to conduct them (for example, stand-alone Microsoft Word-based prescription writers) are not required to conduct the two new transactions, and if they decide not to conduct them, they would incur neither cost nor benefit. However, if they decide to upgrade their entire e-prescribing system to take advantage of the benefits of these new transactions, they would incur costs. However, we have no clear sense of how many entities would fall into this category.

Entities that e-prescribe now using a product that could be upgraded to conduct the two transactions would incur no cost or benefit if they decide not to upgrade. This would also apply to entities that e-prescribe now using a product that can conduct the two transactions using nonstandard (Non NCPDP SCRIPT) formats, but the functionality is not used. Based on our research, this category likely is the one in which most current e-prescribers fall. If they decide to upgrade, they would incur the cost of the upgrade (unless the upgrade is included in their maintenance agreement) and any testing costs, and would incur the benefits of the two transactions.

Entities that e-prescribe now using a product that can conduct the two transactions using nonstandard formats, and who use the transactions would have to upgrade. They would not enjoy all the benefits of the two new transactions since they would have already been performing them in some manner, but definitely would incur cost savings due to the increased interoperability of using the NCPDP SCRIPT standards. In fact, any entity engaging in e-prescribing would incur benefits due to increased interoperability, as the existence of standards simplifies data exchange product selection and testing. We solicit industry and other interested stakeholder comment and input on these issues.

In the e-prescribing final rule at 70 FR 67589, we also discussed the estimated start-up costs for e-prescribing for providers and/or dispensers. Based on industry input, we cited approximately $3,000 for annual support, maintenance, infrastructure and licensing costs. Physicians at that time reported paying user-based licensing fees ranging from $80 to $400 per month. For further discussion of the start-up costs associated with e-prescribing, see the regulatory impact analysis section of this proposed regulation, and the e-prescribing final rule at 70 FR 67589.

In the November 7, 2005 final rule, we addressed the issues of privacy and security relative to e-prescribing in general. We noted that disclosures of protected health information (PHI) in connection with e-prescribing transactions would have to meet the minimum necessary requirements of the Privacy Rule if the entity is a covered entity (70 FR 6161). It is important to note that health plans, prescribers, and dispensers are HIPAA covered entities, and that these covered entities under HIPAA must continue to abide by the applicable HIPAA standards including these for privacy and security.

We continue to agree that privacy and security are important issues related to e-prescribing. Achieving the benefits of e-prescribing require the prescriber and dispenser to have access to patient medical information that may not have been previously available to them.

Section 1860-D (e)(2) (C) of the Act requires that disclosure of patient data in e-prescribing must, at a minimum, comply with HIPAA's privacy and security requirements.

Although HIPAA standards for privacy and security are flexible and scalable to each entity's situation, they provide comprehensive protections. We will continue to evaluate additional standards for consideration as adopted e-prescribing standards. For further discussion of privacy and security and e-prescribing, refer to the final rule at 70 FR 67581 through 67582.

1. Retail Pharmacy

Because e-prescribing is voluntary for pharmacies, dispensers who do not currently conduct e-prescribing would not incur any costs related to any of the provisions of this rule. However, we recognize that costs would be incurred by those dispensers that currently conduct e-prescribing transactions, as well as those who voluntarily implement e-prescribing during the period reflected in our regulatory impact analysis. Industry estimates are that close to 100 percent of the nation's retail chain pharmacies are connected live to an e-prescribing network, with over 95 percent of those connected to networks capable of receiving and exchanging formulary and benefit and medication history data. This is in contrast to only 20 percent of independent pharmacies that are connected to e-prescribing networks.

The transaction using the NCPDP Formulary and Benefit Standard 1.0 is carried out between the plan and prescriber and, therefore, pharmacies will not incur any cost related to this transaction.

While the NCPDP SCRIPT 8.1 Medication History transaction supports communication between the dispenser and prescriber, its use is, nonetheless, voluntary for both. We assume for purposes of this analysis that the Medication History transaction will be carried out between the plan and prescriber, and therefore preliminarily conclude that pharmacies will not incur costs related to this transaction. We solicit industry and other interested stakeholder comment and input on this issue.

The modification of the NCPDP SCRIPT 5.0 foundation standard to NCPDP SCRIPT 8.1 at §423.160(b)(1) will impact pharmacies. Pharmacies will have to assure that their software can accept prescription transactions using the 8.1 standard, and they will need to test with prescribers to assure that their electronic transactions are being received and can be processed. We believe there is little, if any, incremental costs associated with these activities. Software vendors are already implementing version 8.1 in their products, and we believe that any needed upgrades will be included in routine version upgrades. The number of current e-prescribers per pharmacy is small, and the testing process is not complicated. We believe that the implementation of the NPI will be accomplished as part of this transition. Prescribers and dispensers already use the NPI to conduct retail pharmacy drug claim transactions.

2. Medical Practices

Medical practices, compared to pharmacies, face a different set of costs in implementing information systems for clinical care and financial management. Unlike pharmacies, where technology has become an important part of operations (especially for larger retail chains), many providers have been cautious in their adoption of health information technology. We assume that, based on industry estimates, anywhere from 5 to 18 percent of physicians are e-prescribing today (E-Prescribing and the Prescription Drug Program final rule, published November 7, 2005 (70 FR

67568). Because e-prescribing is voluntary for prescribers, medical practices that do not currently conduct e-prescribing would not incur any costs related to any of the provisions of this rule. However, we recognize that costs would be incurred by those prescribers currently e-prescribing, as well as those who voluntarily begin to e-prescribe during the period reflected in our regulatory impact analysis. If a practice decides to implement e-prescribing at a later time, we anticipate that the software products on the market would be compliant with these standards and, therefore, no additional cost would be incurred. In assessing the cost to prescribers that are currently e-prescribing, many of the e-prescribing software products generally already contain some capability to communicate formulary and benefit and medication history information because they incorporate the RxHub proprietary format on which the proposed standards were based. We expect that any changes that might be necessary as a result of this rulemaking would likely be included in routine version upgrades that are covered by annual maintenance and/or subscription fees. We solicit industry and other interested stakeholder comment and input on this issue. For e-prescribers whose software products are not able to generate NCPDP SCRIPT 8.1 transactions, they will not have the capability to conduct the proposed NCPDP Formulary and Benefit Standard 1.0 and NCPDP SCRIPT 8.1 medication history transaction. Costs would be incurred if they were to replace such software with software that generates transactions that comply with the proposed standards. We anticipate that the NCPDP SCRIPT 8.1 will be accommodated in later software version upgrades where that standard is not already utilized. We believe that the implementation of the NPI will be accomplished as part of this transition. Prescribers and dispensers already should be using the NPI to conduct retail pharmacy drug claim transactions.

3. Medicare Part D Plan Sponsors and Pharmacy Benefit Managers (PBMs)
Plan sponsors will be required to support NCPDP SCRIPT 8.1 for the transactions listed at §423.160(b)(1), the NCPDP Formulary and Benefit Standard 1.0, and the NCPDP SCRIPT 8.1 Medication History transaction. They will need to assure that their software can receive and create NCPDP Formulary and Benefit Standard 1.0 and NCPDP SCRIPT 8.1 Medication History transaction queries and responses, and that their internal systems and databases can supply the information needed to build the transaction. For example, they will need to be able to extract prescription claims history and format it according to the Medication History transaction in the NCPDP SCRIPT 8.1 Standard. We believe that many plans

will have already implemented this functionality because the standards we are proposing are based on proprietary file transfer protocols developed by Rx-Hub that have been included in many e-prescribing products. Plans may need to restructure systems to assure that the data output is in the proper format, but, for the most part, the needed functionality is in place.

We recognize that some Medicare Part D plans may need to make additional investments to support these standards, and we solicit industry and other interested stakeholder comment and input on this issue.

Because plans typically pay the per transaction network fees for eligibility transactions, which likely includes providing a formulary and benefit response as well as a medication history response, Medicare Part D plans will incur increased transaction costs for formulary and benefit and medication history transactions as the frequency in which these transactions are conducted electronically increases.

Through information provided by SureScripts and industry consultants, this transaction fee appears to range from 6 cents to 25 cents per transaction, with the midpoint being 15 cents. In 2006, RxHub, one of the nation's largest electronic prescription and prescription-related information routing networks, estimated that their transaction volume increased 50 percent, from 29 million in 2005 to more than 43 million in 2006. These transactions were real-time requests for patient eligibility and benefits, formulary and medication history information (RxHub Announces 2006 e-Prescribing Results and Highlights Milestones for 2007, St. Paul, MN, February 23, 2007, http://www.rxhub.com).

Based on CMS data, we estimate that approximately 24 million Medicare beneficiaries received Medicare Part D benefits in 2006. This figure reflects those Medicare beneficiaries enrolled in a Medicare Prescription Drug Plan (PDP) and/or a Medicare Advantage plan with Prescription Drug coverage (MA-PD), for which CMS has prescription drug event data. Approximately 825,000,000 claims (prescription drug events) were finalized and accepted for 2006 payment.

The annual percentage increase in the number of Medicare Part D prescriptions is estimated by CMS at 4.6 percent based on industry estimates (http://www.imshealth.com/ims/portal/front/articleC/0,2777,6599_3665_80415465, 00.html). So that impact comparisons can be made equally across all years, inflation was removed from the price effects. Conservatively, we calculate the increase in the number of Medicare Part D prescriptions and apply the current estimates of 5 and 18 percent electronic prescribing adoption rates to arrive at the number of Medicare Part D electronic transactions, and cost them out at a range of a low of

6 cents per transaction to a high of 25 cents per transaction. We estimate costs for Medicare Part D plans of between $2 million to $46 million per year.

Medicare Part D plan sponsors may negotiate the cost of e-prescribing transactions as part of the dispensing fees included in their pharmacy contracts, and account for these costs in their annual bids to participate in the Medicare Part D program. In these instances, inclusion of these costs may increase the cost of their Medicare Part D bids. However, we anticipate that these costs would be negated by the savings from an increased rate of conversion from brand name to generic prescriptions realized through utilization of the formulary and benefit transaction, which would more than offset the transaction costs, and solicit comments on this assumption.

4. Vendors

Vendors of e-prescribing software will incur costs to bring their products into compliance with these requirements. However, we consider the need to enhance functionality and comply with industry standards to be a normal cost of doing business that will be subsumed into normal version upgrade activities. Vendors may incur somewhat higher costs connected with testing activities but vendors should be able to address this potential workload on a flow basis. We believe these costs to be minimal, and solicit industry and other interested stakeholder comment and input on this issue.

C. Benefits

The benefits of the proposed adoption of standards for formulary and benefits and medication history transactions take place over a multi-year timeframe. The benefits come in the form of beneficiary cost savings realized by increases in formulary adherence and/or generic versus brand name prescribing by physicians as a result of realtime access to formulary and benefits information, administrative (time and labor cost) savings through reduced call-backs on the part of both physicians and pharmacists, and a reduction of the occurrence of preventable adverse drug events (ADEs) among Medicare beneficiaries, reducing resultant health care costs.

1. Formulary and Benefit Standard—Generic Drug Usage

We assume that, based on industry estimates, approximately 5 percent to 18 percent of group practices are e-prescribing today, and use that range for our assumptions. The formulary and benefit transaction will allow the prescriber to view formulary drugs, alternative preferred drugs in a given class that may offer savings to the patient, and/or to see in advance what other less costly drugs within a given drug classification and/or generic drugs can be substituted for a given brand name prescription drug. This can result in reducing calls to the plan, and/or reducing the number of callbacks from a pharmacy because a prescribed drug is not on a beneficiary's drug plan formulary.

In 2006, 60 percent of Medicare Part D prescriptions in the first two quarters of the program were for generic drugs, and the remaining 40 percent were brand name prescription drugs. During a Medco study of physicians using e-prescribing technology (http://medco.mediaroom.com/index.php?s=43&item=100), physicians increased their generic substitution rates by over 15 percent. However, we recognize that not all beneficiaries will accept generic prescription drugs and there are some instances, especially when prescribing for mental health conditions, in which the brand name prescription drug has proven through physician experience to be the more effective drug, and therefore the drug of choice. Therefore, we apply a more conservative 7 percent annual increase in generic prescriptions.

We again apply the previously used 5 and 18 percent e-prescribing estimate range. Based on industry data, we assume the cost of a brand name prescription drug at $111.02 and the cost of a generic drug at $32.23. (http://www.nacds.org/wmspage.cfm?parm1=5507. National Association of Chain Drug Stores data.)

While Medicare beneficiaries will be the most direct recipients of the benefit realized by the conversion of brand name to generic prescription drugs, the Medicare program will benefit as well. The Medicare program will save money as it will be paying for an increased number of lower-cost generic prescriptions versus higher-cost, brandname prescription drugs. We calculate a cost savings of $95 million to $410 million.

2. Formulary and Benefit Standard—Administrative Savings

a. Physician and Physician Office Staff

The 2004 Medical Group Management Association (MGMA) survey entitled, "Analyzing the Cost of Administrative Complexity" (http://www.mgma.com/about/default.aspx?id=280) estimated the staff and physician time spent, on a per physician full time equivalent (FTE) basis, interacting with pharmacies on formulary questions and generic substitutions. Physician time on the phone discussing formulary issues was estimated at almost 16 hours a year; another 14 hours were spent per physician per year on generic substitution issues. Staff spent almost 26 hours per FTE physician on formulary issues, and another 24 hours per FTE physician on generic substitution issues.

CMS estimates the number of physicians in active practice who participated in the Medicare program in 2006 at 1,048,2436 (2006 CMS Statistics, U.S. Department of Health and Human Services CMS Pub. No. 03470, July 2006, Table 22).

Based on the same CMS data from 2003 through 2006, it indicates a percentage rise in the number of physicians participating in the Medicare program of .94 percent per year, so we have applied that percentage increase to arrive at an estimated number of Medicare physicians for 2009 through 2013. We also apply the previous assumption that from 5 to 18 percent of prescribers are e-prescribing today. Per the MGMA survey, we assume a physician labor cost of $100 per hour and an average staff labor cost of $22 per hour per physician FTE.

Pilot site experience shows that, among prescribers or their agents who adopted e-prescribing, obtaining prior approvals, responding to refill requests, and resolving pharmacy callbacks were all done more efficiently with e-prescribing than before. Both groups perceived a greater than 50 percent reduction in time to manage refill requests and significant time savings in managing pharmacy call backs (Findings from the Evaluation of E-Prescribing Pilot Sites, http://www.healthit.ahrq.gov.) However, we are realistic in our assumption that full implementation would be difficult to achieve, and use an estimate of 25 percent. Our model calculates that physicians and staff would realize savings ranging from $55 million to $206 million at a 25 percent implementation rate.

b. Pharmacists

If each physician and their office staff save a total of 80 hours a year by using the formulary and benefit transaction and reducing the time spent on the phone with pharmacists, we assume that pharmacists are saving the equivalent amount of time by not making these calls. Since the MGMA survey assumes a pharmacist labor rate of $60 per hour, our model predicts that, at an annualized cost savings, pharmacists would realize an annualized cost benefit savings ranging from a low of $65 million to a high of $242 million at 25 percent implementation.

3. Medication History Standard—Reduction of Adverse Drug Events (ADEs)

Automating the transmission of medication history information will simplify medication reconciliation through transitions in care and, in so doing, provide a safer and more effective health care system. Consumers will benefit from a safer medication delivery system, and greater convenience.

Although outpatient ADEs are difficult to estimate, current literature estimates that, as of 2005, there were 530,000 preventable ADEs for Medicare beneficiaries (Field TS, Gilman BH, Subramanian S, Fuller JC, Bates DW, Gurwitz JH. 2005. The costs associated with adverse drug events among older adults in the ambulatory setting. *Medical Care* 43(12):1171–1176.) Moreover, the estimated cost per ADE ranges from $2,000 (Field TS, Gilman BH, Subramanian S, Fuller JC, Bates DW, Gurwitz JH. 2005. The costs associated with adverse drug events among older adults in the ambulatory setting. *Medical Care* 43(12):1171–1176.) to upwards of $6,000 (Institute of Medicine of the National Academies. Preventing Medication Errors. July, 2006. Field TS, Gilman BH, Subramanian S, Fuller JC, Bates DW, Gurwitz JH. 2005.) The costs associated with adverse drug events among older adults in the ambulatory setting. *Medical Care* 43(12):1171–1176. (Field TS, Gilman BH, Subramanian S, Fuller JC, Bates DW, Gurwitz JH. 2005. The costs associated with adverse drug events among older adults in the ambulatory setting. *Medical Care* 43(12):1171–1176.) depending on the care setting. We chose to compute the benefits of medication history based on ADEs as a percentage of the total Medicare population. Based on CMS data from 1999 through 2006, the total Medicare population increased on average 1.13 percent per year (2006 CMS Statistics, U.S. Department of Health and Human Services CMS Pub. No. 03470, July 2006, Table 1). We calculated that of the total Medicare population, ADEs occur in about 1.24 percent of that population each year.

Brigham and Women's Hospital discovered in their analysis of ADEs, conducted as part of the CMS e-prescribing pilot project, that e-prescribing could reduce the risk of ADEs by approximately 50 percent. (Findings from the Evaluation of E-Prescribing Pilot Sites, http://www.healthit.ahrq.gov) As medication history is a transaction that most directly impacts ADEs (versus formulary and benefit, codified SIG, etc.), we assume that the reduction in the risk of ADEs can be attributed mostly to the use of medication history rather than to e-prescribing in general. The pilot project demonstrated that 50 percent of preventable ADEs could be eliminated via e-prescribing, and possibly more as prescriber familiarity with the medication history function and full clinical decision support tools become available in all e-prescribing software. We also recognize that the Brigham and Women's Hospital ADE analysis brings with it a degree of uncertainty, as it was a by-product of the pilot project itself, and may not accurately represent the experiences of all entities (that is, small rural settings). Given that, we conservatively assume that the number of ambulatory ADEs associated with Medicare Part D beneficiaries could be reduced by 25 percent for the proportion of patients for whom prescriptions are written electronically; we use the same uptake e-prescribing estimates (5 to 18 percent) as earlier for e-prescribing adoption.

The introduction of e-prescribing can potentially realize a cost savings of $13 million to $156 million from avoided ADEs. We solicit industry and other interested stakeholder comment and input on this issue. Besides lower rates of ADEs, the public will also realize other benefits related to the medication history function of e-prescribing. Through improved collaboration and communication between physicians and plans, patients will be more likely to have greater access to information which will encourage them to become more involved in their own treatment, which studies show decreases the probability of experiencing an ADE-related error.[8]

C. Total Impact

This analysis has focused on the costs and benefits of two new e-prescribing standards, and the adoption of NCPDP SCRIPT 8.1 in place of version 5.0. We conclude that the cost of implementing these proposals is minimal, with quantifiable benefits reaped by pharmacies, providers, and beneficiaries. Over time, we expect that these groups will see average benefits in a range from $218.0 million to $863.9 million from the utilization of formulary and benefit and medication history transactions and the promulgation of these standards (Table 6).

Part 423—Voluntary Medicare Prescription Drug Benefit: §423.160 Standards for Electronic Prescribing

Standards

(1) Prescription

The National Council for the Prescription Drug Programs Prescriber/Pharmacist Interface SCRIPT Standard, Implementation Guide Version 8, Release 1 (Version 8.1), October 2005 to provide for the communication of a prescription or prescription-related information between prescribers and dispensers, for the following:

    i. Get message transaction.
    ii. Status response transaction.
    iii. Error response transaction.

iv. New prescription transaction.

v. Prescription change request transaction.

vi. Prescription change response transaction.

vii. Refill prescription request transaction.

viii. Refill prescription response transaction.

ix. Verification transaction.

x. Password change transaction.

xi. Cancel prescription request transaction.

xii. Cancel prescription response transaction.

(2)

* * *

(3) Medication history

The National Council for Prescription Drug Programs (NCPDP) Prescriber/ Pharmacist Interface SCRIPT Standard, Implementation Guide, Version 8, Release 1 (Version 8.1), October 2005 to provide for the communication of Medicare Part D medication history information among Medicare Part D sponsors, prescribers, and dispensers.

(4) Formulary and benefits

The National Council for Prescription Drug Programs (NCPDP) Formulary and Benefits Standard, Implementation Guide, Version 1, Release 0 (Version 1.0), October 2005 for transmitting formulary and benefit information between prescribers and Medicare Part D sponsors.

(5) Provider identifier

The National Provider Identifier (NPI), as defined at 45 CFR 162.406, to identify a health care provider in Medicare Part D e-prescribing or prescription-related transactions conducted among Medicare Part D plan sponsors, prescribers, and dispensers when a health care provider's identifier is required.

GLOSSARY

AHIC   American Health Information Community.

AHIMA   American Health Information Management Association.

AHRQ   Agency for Healthcare Research and Quality.

ANSI   American National Standards Institute.

ASTHO   Association of State and Territorial Health Officials.

Accredited Standards Committee (ASC)   *See* X12N 270/271.

Adverse Drug Events (ADEs)   Any injury due to medication (e.g., drowsiness from chlorpheniramine).

Adverse Drug Reaction (ADR)   *See* ADE.

American National Standards Institute (ANSI)   A private nonprofit federation that includes industry; standards development organizations; trade associations; professional and technical societies; government; and labor and consumer groups. It serves as a forum for public and private sector cooperative development of voluntary national consensus standards.

BSV   Biosurveillance.

Beer's List   A national guideline and reference guide for pharmacists and physicians to improve the use of medication in seniors, developed with explicit criteria based on the risk–benefit definition of appropriateness and originally with the frail elderly nursing facility resident in mind. It now has been revised several times and has an ambulatory focus as well.

CC   Chronic Care.

CDC   Centers for Disease Control and Prevention.

CDISC   Clinical Data Interchange Standards Consortium.

CE   Consumer Empowerment.

CHI   Consolidated Health Informatics.

CCHIT   Certification Commission for Healthcare Information Technology.

CDS   Clinical Decision Support.

CHC   Community Health Centers.

CMS   Centers for Medicare and Medicaid Services.

CPRS   Computerized Patient Record System.

DEA   U.S. Federal Drug Enforcement Administration.

DoD   Department of Defense.

Dispenser   A person or other legal entity licensed, registered, or otherwise permitted by the jurisdiction in which the person practices or the entity is located to provide drug products for human use by prescription in the course of professional practice.

e-Refills   The ability to use e-prescribing systems to OK and/or monitor refill prescriptions.

EDI   Electronic data interchange.

EHR   Electronic health record.

EMR   Electronic medical record (same as EHR).

EHRVA   Electronic Health Record Vendors Association.

FACA   Federal Advisory Committee Act.

FDA   Food and Drug Administration.

FHA   Federal Health Architecture.

FORE   Foundation of Research and Education (part of AHMA; works for ONC).

Fill Status   Informs when Rx is filled, not filled, or partially filled; includes provider, patient, and drug segments of SCRIPT message; not yet generally used.

Final Standards   Uniform standards that are adopted through notice and comment rule making for use in the e-prescribing program under Title I of the MMA. Medicare prescription drug program sponsors, Medicare Advantage (MA) organizations offering Medicare Advantage-Prescription Drug (MA-PD) plans, and other Part D sponsors will be required to support and comply with these standards when electronically transmitting prescriptions and prescription-related information between dispensing pharmacies and pharmacists.

Formulary and Benefit Information   This standard displays the formulary (a list of drugs covered by a plan) status and alternative drugs as well as co-pays and other status information.

Foundation Standards   Standards for which there is adequate industry experience that have been adopted by DHHS Secretary through notice and comment rule making without pilot testing.

HHS   U.S. Department of Health and Human Services.

HIE   Health information exchange.

HIMSS   Healthcare Information Management Systems Society.

HIPAA   Health Insurance Portability and Accountability Act.

HISB   Healthcare Informatics Standards Board.

HISPC   Health Information Security and Privacy.

HIT   Health information technology.

HITPC   Health Information Technology Policy Council.

HITSP   Health Information Technology Standards Panel.

HL7   Health level 7.

HRSA   Health Resources and Services Administration.

IFMC   Iowa Foundation for Medical Informatics.

IHS   Indian Health Service.

IOM   Institute of Medicine.

IT   Information technology.

Initial Standards   Standards that NCVHS reviewed and commented on, which were ultimately recognized by the Secretary as initial uniform standards relating to the requirements for e-prescribing. These standards lacked adequate industry experience and thus were subject to pilot testing via the AHRQ interagency agreement with CMS.

JCAHO   Joint Commission on Accreditation of Health Care Organizations. *See* TJC.

MUA   Medically underserved areas.

Medicare Advantage (MA) Organizations   A public or private entity organized and licensed by a state as a risk-bearing entity that is certified by CMS as meeting the MA contract requirements.

Medicare Advantage Plan   A type of Medicare plan offered by a private company that contracts with Medicare to provide Medicare Part A and Part B benefits; also called Part C.

Medicare Advantage Prescription Drug Plans (MA-PDs)   A Medicare Advantage plan that provides qualified prescription drug coverage under Part D of Title XVIII of the Social Security Act.

Medicare Prescription Drug Plan (PDP)   A stand-alone plan that only offers prescription drug coverage under Part D of Title XVIII of the Social Security Act.

Medication Error   Any error occurring in the medication use process; includes preventable, inappropriate use of medication, such as prescribing, dispensing, and administering.

Medication History (Hx)   Standard that includes the status, provider, patient, coordination of benefit, repeatable drug, request, and response segments of SCRIPT.

NAHIT   National Alliance for Health Information Technology; the Alliance.

NCI   National Cancer Institute.

NCPDP (National Council for Prescription Drug Programs)   A not-for-profit ANSI-accredited Standards Development Organization that develops and maintains standards through a consensus building process among more than 1,450 members representing all pharmacy sectors.

NCPDP Provider Identifier Number   Widely accepted as the dispenser (pharmacy) identifier (there is currently no single identifier required for prescribers). Its database contains information to support various claims processing functions.

NCPDP SCRIPT Cancellation   Cancels a prescription previously sent to a pharmacy.

NCPDP SCRIPT Change Request and Response   The primary means by which a pharmacy may request of a provider a clarification, correction, or change in drug as a result of therapeutic substitution or other rationale.

NCPDP SCRIPT Fill Status   *See* Fill Status.

NCPDP SCRIPT Formulary and Benefit Information   *See* Formulary and Benefit Information.

NCPDP SCRIPT Medication History   *See* Medication History.

NCPDP SCRIPT Standard   Provides for the exchange of new prescriptions, changes, renewals, cancellations, and Fill Status notifications. The NCPDP SCRIPT Standard supports a wide variety of transactions, from new prescriptions to refill requests, prescription change responses to fill status notification.

NCPDP Telecommunication Standard   The HIPAA standard for eligibility communications between retail pharmacy dispensers and payers/PBMs.

NCSL   National Conference of State Legislatures.

NCVHS   National Committee on Vital and Health Statistics.

NGA   National Governors Association.

NHIN   Nationwide Health Information Network.

NIH   National Institutes of Health.

NLM   National Library of Medicine.

OCSQ   Office of Clinical Standards and Quality.

OHITA   Office of Health Information Technology Adoption.

OIS   Office of Interoperability and Standards.

OMB   Office of Management and Budget.

ONC   Office of the National Coordinator (preferred abbreviation for ONCHIT).

ONCHIT   Office of the National Coordinator for Health Information Technology.

OPC   Office of Programs and Coordination.

OPR   Office of Policy and Research.

PARTner IFMC's system for collecting data from everyone who reports data in to OCSQ.

PHC Personalized health care.

PHCCC Population Health & Clinical Care Connections.

PHR Personal health record.

PITAC President's Information Technology Advisory Committee.

PQRI Physician Quality Reporting Initiative.

PVRP Physician Voluntary Reporting Program.

Part D Sponsors Private organizations that contract with Medicare to offer prescription drug insurance plans under Part D of Title XVIII of the Social Security Act.

Pharmacy Benefits Managers (PBMs) Private companies that administer pharmacy benefits and manage the purchasing, dispensing, and reimbursing of prescription drugs. PBMs provide a wide array of services to health insurers or to large health care purchasers and may negotiate rebates or discounts from pharmaceutical manufacturers and retail pharmacies and process claims for prescription drugs. PBMs play a key role in managing pharmacy benefit plans in the Medicare drug program.

Practice Management System (PMS) Tools (usually computer software) that organize routine medical and business tasks.

Prior Authorization The portion of X12N 278 standard that supports prior authorization. It requires header information, requester, subscriber, utilization management, and other relevant information.

Prescriber A physician, dentist, or other person licensed, registered, or otherwise permitted by the United States or the jurisdiction in which he or she practices to issue prescriptions for drugs for human use.

QUAL Quality.

RHIO Regional Health Information Network.

RPMS Resource and Patient Management System.

RTF Review Task Force.

RxNorm A clinical drug nomenclature produced by the NLM that provides standard names for clinical drugs and for dose forms and links from clinical drugs to their active ingredients, drug components, and most related brand names. It includes the semantic clinical drug (ingredient plus strength and dose form) and the semantic branded drug representation (proprietary, branded ingredient plus strength).

SAMHSA Substance Abuse and Mental Health Services Administration.

SNOMED Systematized Nomenclature of Medicine.

Schedule II Drugs A drug or chemical substance whose possession and use are regulated under the Controlled Substances Act, including, among others, narcotics and hallucinogens.

SIG Messages indication, dose, dose calculation, dose restriction, route, frequency, interval, site, administration time, and duration.

TJC The Joint Commission. Formerly known as JCAHO; the commission shortened its name in 2007.

VHA Veterans Health Administration.

VISTA Veterans Health Information Systems and Technology Architecture.

VOE Vista Office EHR.

WG Work group.

X12N 270/271 The HIPAA standard for eligibility and benefits communications between dentists, professionals, institutions, and health plans.

X12N 278 *See* prior authorization.

INDEX